NEW REPRODUCTIVE TECHNIQUES

NEW REPRODUCTIVE TECHNIQUES
A Legal Perspective

DOUGLAS J. CUSINE
University of Aberdeen

Gower

Aldershot · Brookfield USA · Hong Kong · Singapore · Sydney

Published by
Gower Publishing Company Limited
Gower House
Croft Road
Aldershot
Hants GU11 3HR
England

Gower Publishing Company
Old Post Road
Brookfield
Vermont 05036
USA

British Library Cataloguing in Publication Data

Cusine, Douglas J., *1946–*
    New reproductive techniques: a legal
    perspective.—(Medico-legal issues;
    v. 10).
    1. Great Britain. Man. Reproduction
    scientific innovation. Legal aspects
    I. Title II. Series
    342.104'419

Library of Congress Cataloging-in-Publication Data

Cusine, Douglas J.
    New reproductive techniques: a legal perspective/Douglas J.
    Cusine.
        p.   cm.—(Medico-legal issues; v. 10)
    Bibliography: p.
    Includes index.
    ISBN 0–566–05410–8: £25.00 ($50.00 U.S.)
    1. Artificial insemination, Human—Law and legislation—Great
    Britain.   2. Fertilization in vitro, Human—Law and legislation—
    Great Britain.   I. Title.   II. Series.
    KD3415.C87 1988
    344.41'0419—dc19
    [344. 104419]

    ISBN 0 566 05410 8

Printed and bound in Great Britain by
Anchor Brendon Ltd, Tiptree, Essex

Contents

CONTENTS

Foreword

Since the introduction of *in vitro* fertilization in 1978 when the first child conceived by this technique was born, the subject of infertility has been much more widely discussed than before. New techniques of treating this complaint have been introduced and the outlook for a couple with infertility problems is now much more hopeful than it was two decades ago. Much research effort has gone into perfecting these methods but a great deal more needs to be done in the future to make the success rate better than it is at present. For example, each woman who undergoes *in vitro* fertilization has about a 1 in 10 chance of having a baby in the end.

The new techniques have meant that for the first time conception can occur outside the human body. This has posed society with very complex ethical and legal problems. What is the status of a human embryo; does it deserve the same respect as a child or an adult; what should be done with 'spare' embryos; should experimentation be allowed on human embryos? Should 'the law' be introduced into this area of treatment? The Warnock Committee sat for two years and published its Report. A number of recommendations were made, some of which required that legislation be enacted so that there were restrictions on what could and could not be done in this field.

Three years later parliament has produced only one piece of legislation as a result of the Report, namely the Surrogacy Arrangements Act 1985, which outlaws commercial surrogacy and bans advertising about it. However a consultative document has been issued on all aspects of the new infertility treatments and a white paper at the end of 1987, so new legislation can be expected on this subject.

To a lay person it does not appear that it should be too difficult to legislate for some of the problems. For example, the Warnock Committee suggested that the AID child should be legitimate if the husband agreed to his wife being inseminated by donor. However, as this book suggests, there are numerous complications from the legal point of view and many ramifications regarding this suggestion. If the husband does not agree and the wife goes ahead with insemination – is the child illegitimate?

What has struck me reading this book are the immensely complicated legal issues that are involved. Douglas Cusine is to be congratulated on putting all these down before us so that we can understand the complexity of the issues and how carefully they must be examined before legislation is introduced. One contentious issue is – who is the child's mother when the carrying mother makes no genetic contribution to the child, that is, the gametes come from a husband and wife and the embryo is implanted into a third person. When we contemplate saying that the woman who gives birth to the child may not be its mother, matters become very complicated indeed. The legal status of a child born to a surrogate is much more complex than it first seems and this book explores this in depth. I would suggest that all Members of both Houses of Parliament should read this book before any debate on legislation for artificial reproduction. It sets out in a clear way the complex legal issues with their theological, moral, social and scientific implications and it should be of great help to anyone who is trying to determine what to do regarding legislation.

The ultimate objective should be for the legislation introduced to make society, as far as this area is concerned, one which in the words of the Warnock Report we can 'praise and admire', a society in which we can live with a clear conscience. This book should help us to do this.

Sir Malcolm Macnaughton

Preface

I first became interested in the legal issues raised by the modern reproductive techniques when I read a commentary in *New Scientist* in the early 1970s. It prompted me to write a few articles in which I attempted to analyze these issues, especially those surrounding artificial insemination by donor. Shortly after their publication I was fortunate to be invited to participate in the Fourth Study Group of the Royal College of Obstetricians and Gynaecologists. Those present, and others, stimulated my interest and I have benefited enormously from my contact with them. Included among them are Charles Butcher, Georges David, Gordon Dunstan, Robert Edwards, Max Elstein, Arnold Klopper, Harry Krause, John Loudon, Callum Macnaughton, John McNeil, Ken Mason, David Richardson, Eddie Smith and Allan Templeton.

I am particularly grateful to Arnold Klopper and his wife Mary. I have had a most enjoyable and rewarding association with Arnold over the years. Both he and Mary read an earlier draft of the manuscript and for that, and their many other kindnesses over the years, I owe them a great deal.

I am also indebted to Callum Macnaughton, President of the Royal College of Obstetricians and Gynaecologists. I have benefited immensely from our many discussions and I am particularly pleased that, despite a very full schedule, he has provided the Foreword for this book, a gesture of his kindness which is much appreciated.

Russell Scott, the Chairman of the Australian Law Reform Commission, provided me with valuable material on the legal position in Australia which assisted me greatly and saved a substantial amount of time.

Sheila McLean, General Editor of the series in which this book appears, read a draft of the manuscript and made many suggestions for its improvement. For that, and her continued support throughout the gestation period, I have much reason to be thankful.

My head of department, Phil Love, encouraged me to pursue my interest in this area which has little or nothing to do with the Scots

Law of Conveyancing. Wearing one of his many other hats, he too is now very involved in these developments!

I have attempted to produce a book which will assist those who are involved and interested in the modern reproductive techniques and the associated legal issues, whether as obstetrician, researcher, legal adviser or whatever. If I have provided something which might help to solve a problem, or merely identify one, then that is due in no small measure to all – including those already mentioned – who have given me their advice and assistance. If I have failed it is despite their efforts.

Douglas J. Cusine
Aberdeen, December 1987

Abbreviations

ABAJ	*American Bar Association Journal*
AI	artificial insemination
AID	AI with semen from a donor
AIH	AI using the husband's semen
BMA	British Medical Association
BMJ	*British Medical Journal*
Fert. & Ster.	*Fertility and Sterility*
IPPF	International Planned Parenthood Federation
IVF	*in vitro* fertilization
JAMA	*Journal of the American Medical Association*
J. For. Med.	*Journal of Forensic Medicine*
J. Med. Eth.	*Journal of Medical Ethics*
MRC	Medical Research Council
NEJM	*New England Journal of Medicine*
NLJ	*New Law Journal*
NYULR	*New York University Law Report*
RCOG	Royal College of Obstetrics and Gynaecology
SALJ	*South African Law Journal*
U. Fla. LR	*University of Florida Law Report*

PART I
INTRODUCTION

1 Introduction

In the past, couples who were unable to have children probably had to accept their childless state as an irreversible condition. This was because medical science had not identified many of the causes of infertility and hence could not provide remedies.

Human artificial insemination using the husband's semen (AIH) was first practised at the end of the eighteenth century, but it was probably not until the present century that it was practised widely or that it became generally known. The nineteenth century saw the use of artificial insemination with semen from a donor (AID), but it has been developed only in the last forty years. If neither of these techniques is known to the couple or acceptable to them they might be able to adopt a child, but that would not satisfy a desire to have their own child and with the increased availability of contraception and abortion there are fewer children for adoption.

However, since 1960 AI services have improved and the technique has become more acceptable to the public in general. In many centres semen is stored for long periods by freezing it (cryopreservation), and so it can be available to the woman at the best possible time.

Artificial insemination is a solution where the reason for the childlessness is the man's infertility, or because it would be inadvisable for him to father a child. Where it is the woman who cannot, or would be advised not to have a child other solutions are available. These include egg (ovum) donation which is the counterpart to AID, and *in vitro* fertilization (IVF). The latter was developed over a period of years by Robert Edwards and Patrick Steptoe and culminated in the birth of a child – the first 'test-tube baby' – in 1978. This possibility of fertilizing an egg outside the woman's body means that the resulting embryo or embryos can be implanted into another woman (embryo transfer) where, for example, both she and her husband are infertile. The resulting child would have two mothers and two fathers. The two mothers are the genetic mother who produced the egg and the nurturing mother in whose body the embryo develops into a baby, and there is the genetic father and the nurturing 'father' who will bring the child up as his own.

There is another situation in which a child may have two mothers and possibly two fathers and that is where a woman has agreed to bear a child for someone else. This is known as surrogacy of which there are a number of permutations (see Appendix), but the child may still have a genetic mother and a nurturing mother who are different people.

Human semen is normally preserved in connection with AID, but a husband's semen could be preserved for a number of reasons, and a woman could therefore conceive a child by her husband after his death. Cryopreservation has been extended to embryos and more recently to human eggs. The embryos which are frozen are those which have not been implanted into a woman, but instead of being preserved, they could be used for research into such things as inheritable diseases. That raises the issue of the status of these embryos, the extent to which research may be carried out and the type of research.

The main use of artificial insemination and the other techniques has been to alleviate infertility. However AID has also been employed to avoid the transmission of an inheritable disease, and egg donation, embryo transfer etc. could also be used for this.

The ensuing chapters look at the legal issues which arise from the use of these techniques and examine them chiefly in connection with the alleviation of infertility. The wider implications however are not to be ignored.

2 Infertility: causes and cures

It is impossible to be completely sure how prevalent infertility is. Some couples make a deliberate decision that they are not going to have children; others who would wish to have children decide not to for a variety of reasons. For example, they may think that their accommodation is unsuitable or their income inadequate, or that the world is not a suitable place in which to rear children. Nevertheless it is frequently estimated that somewhere between 10 and 15 per cent of all marriages are infertile.[1] If that figure is even approximately accurate, in any one year there will be between 200 000 and 300 000 married couples in the United States who are involuntarily childless, and between 40 000 and 60 000 in the United Kingdom.[2] These figures do not include cohabiting couples, on whom there is no published information.

Before considering the causes of infertility and possible solutions it is useful to indicate how a pregnancy is usually achieved. Each month an egg is discharged from the ovary and it enters the Fallopian tube which leads to the uterus (womb) and fertilization usually takes place in the tube. Sperm which have been discharged into the vagina make their way into the uterus and into the tube. If an egg has recently ripened it may be fertilized by one of the sperm. The fertilized egg gradually descends and implants itself into the wall of the uterus where it develops into a foetus and, eventually, a child may be born.

There are many reasons why any of these processes may not take place but our concern here is only with infertility.

Causes of infertility

Many factors give rise to infertility but for convenience they can be classified as environmental, physical or psychological. In some cases there is a combination of factors.

In the past it may have been assumed that the woman was

responsible for the infertility. While this view would no longer be supported by the medical profession it is still true to say that greater emphasis has been put on female, rather than male infertility. The cause of the infertility may lie exclusively in the male or the female: in many instances there are factors affecting both which result in their union being childless. Both parties may therefore have to be examined to reveal the cause or causes which, in turn, may determine the solutions.[3] What follows is a brief outline of some of the factors which may affect the male, then those which may affect the female, and finally factors which may affect both. It is important to bear in mind, however, that the reason why a couple cannot have children may not be ascertainable; in other words all the possible causes known to medical science may have been eliminated, but nevertheless the woman still does not conceive. Further details on the causes of infertility can be obtained from specialist works.[4]

The male

An investigation of an infertile couple will usually commence with an analysis of the semen. If the male can sustain an erection and produce semen (an ejaculate), he will generally have no doubt about his virility. It may not therefore occur to him, and he may be unwilling to accept, that he is infertile, that is, the quality of his sperm is not good enough to father children.

To achieve fertilization the male must produce an adequate number of sperm which are moving and of normal shape and size and he must also be capable of depositing these into his partner's vagina. The average ejaculate contains between 60 and 150 million sperm per millilitre, of which about 20 per cent will be abnormal in shape or size or will not move, but the remainder will provide at least the potential for fertilization. However if the male is unable to produce sperm (failure of spermatogenesis) or produces an inadequate number, or the sperm is of poor quality or he is unable to deliver them into the vagina, fertilization is unlikely to occur.

Conditions such as endocrine disorders, stress, disease or structural defects (or even close fitting underwear or having a hot bath, both of which raise the temperature of the scrotal sac) may result in a decrease in sperm production (oligospermia). It is generally accepted that a sperm count of less than 30 million per millilitre means that the man is sub-fertile.[5] More serious conditions resulting in sterility are azoospermia which is the complete absence of sperm, aspermia, the absence of living sperm, and necrospermia, where the sperm are dead.

An absence of, or obstruction in, the ducts leading from the testicles, where the sperm are produced, to the penis may result in infertility because the sperm is not being transported. An obstruction of these ducts commonly results from diseases such as mumps, tuberculosis or gonorrhoea, but the ducts may have been blocked deliberately, in a vasectomy.

Even though the sperm is being produced and transported, it may not be delivered into the vagina. The cause may simply be faulty coital technique, but the male may suffer from premature or retrograde ejaculation or he may be impotent. Any examination of the male therefore will have these factors in mind, but if the male produces a normal ejaculate and he can deposit this into the vagina, attention may turn to his partner.

The female

The examination of the woman will attempt to ascertain three things:

(a) whether she is ovulating, that is, whether eggs are being produced and released from the ovaries through the Fallopian tubes;
(b) whether the genital passages contain any obstruction which would prevent the sperm from getting through to the tubes;
(c) whether the uterus and its lining (the endometrium) are suitable for the implantation and development of a fertilized egg.

A failure to produce eggs may be because the ovary has exhausted its supply. This happens to every female at the menopause – usually around the age of fifty – but occasionally there may be premature ovarian failure, perhaps through disease. Gonorrhoea may result in the non-production of eggs or a blockage of the Fallopian tubes. If there is an obstruction in the genital tract the sperm may be unable to pass through the neck of the womb (cervix).

An actual obstruction of the cervix is rare, but what more commonly prevents sperm transport is the presence in the vagina of fluid which makes it more difficult than usual for sperm to penetrate (hostile cervical mucus). This may have been caused by infection. Infertility may also result if the uterus is abnormally sited or is adversely affected in some way, for example by fibrous tissue. The absence of a uterus clearly means that the woman cannot bear children. However if there is no apparent defect in either the male or the female, then the cause may lie with the couple.

The couple

In some cases both the man and the woman may have been examined and there may not seem to be anything which prevents either of them from having children. However it would be a mistake not to consider the couple as a unit, for there are a number of factors which can affect them as a couple which separate examinations would not necessarily disclose. It is therefore essential at the outset of the investigation to discuss the couple's sexual activities with them. Such discussions may disclose that they are ignorant of the physiology of reproduction, but what is perhaps more likely is that there is something which renders the man impotent with that particular woman, but not necessarily with others, or the woman may not be able to have intercourse with that particular man, although again not necessarily with others. Some women suffer from a contraction of the vaginal muscles (vaginismus) which makes intercourse painful or impossible.

These are the main factors which can result in a couple being childless. It is now appropriate to look at possible solutions.

Solutions to infertility

If a couple find that their union is infertile there are a number of courses open to them. These are (a) to remain childless; (b) for either or both partners to have intercourse with someone else with a view to having a child and bringing it up as their child; (c) to adopt or foster a child; and (d) to take some other measures, which usually involve obtaining medical advice and treatment.

Only the last of these solutions is the subject of this book, but the first three will be considered briefly, as will possible objections to them.

Childlessness

The decision to remain childless does not of itself give rise to legal problems, but it may not be acceptable to the couple. They may feel a need to have children or to create a new generation, or there may be family or social pressures on them to reproduce. Failure to have children may leave them with a feeling of inadequacy and result in marital breakdown or dissolution of the union.[6]

Intercourse with a third party

The second possibility is for either or both partners to have sexual intercourse with someone else. Adultery is a major cause of divorce and if the child is conceived in this way it will often be rejected by the other partner. It may also suffer a social stigma because of the circumstances in which it was conceived. Adultery does, of course, have legal consequences (for example, the child is illegitimate) but these are not considered at great length here for two reasons. The first is that the legal issues are not peculiar to infertility, and secondly they are more appropriately dealt with in specialist books on family law.[7] Having said that, adultery will be mentioned from time to time, particularly in the context of AID, where there has been some discussion as to whether or not it amounts in law to adultery.

Adoption and fostering

The reasons which have just been put forward for the brief treatment of adultery apply equally to adoption and fostering. Adoption is usually the last resort for a childless couple, because there are a number of drawbacks. The most important of these is the acute shortage of children available for adoption. In some places there may be only older or handicapped children. There are however a number of other factors which may make adoption a less welcome solution.

In the first place it can be a lengthy process. In the UK it is not possible to adopt a child until it is at least nineteen weeks old[8] and it may take some months for the process to be completed. Until that comes about the natural parent(s) may decide against adoption and this creates uncertainty for the adopting parents. Secondly the identity of the natural parents will not usually be known to the adopting couple and they may therefore have doubts about the child's background, especially if neither of them has a genetic link with the child. In such a case the couple will be completely unaware of the child's genetic background and it may have inherited some genetic traits to its detriment. Another reason why adoption may not appeal to a childless couple is that they may be slightly older before they find out that they cannot have children and may therefore be regarded as less suitable. Furthermore in the UK an unmarried couple cannot make a joint application to adopt a child.[9]

Fostering a child may have even less appeal for a childless couple. Although it is not as lengthy a process as adoption it is open to some of the objections which have just been mentioned, for example the uncertainty about the child's background. However there are other features which may make it unattractive to a couple who wish to have children of their own. For example, it is not a permanent arrangement and perhaps because of that it may cause both the couple and the child grief when it comes to an end.

Each of these 'solutions' is open to objection and so it is necessary to consider those which involve medical advice and treatment.

Medical advice and treatment

Some of the causes of infertility require nothing more by way of cure than medical advice. That should be all that is required to correct faulty coital technique, or to prevent a man from wearing underwear which is too tight or having a hot bath before inter-course. For some conditions, however, medical treatment is necessary. Surgery will be required to reverse a vasectomy or to remove a blockage in the Fallopian tubes, while drugs may have to be used to remedy a hormonal deficiency or malfunction. These forms of treatment undoubtedly have legal implications, but there are no legal issues which are peculiar to their use in alleviating infertility, and for that reason they are not dealt with here. We shall be concerned only with the legal implications of forms of treatment which are used exclusively, or almost exclusively, in connection with infertility. These are artificial insemination, *in vitro* fertilization, egg donation, embryo transfer and surrogacy.

It is proposed to look at these topics in greater depth, but before doing so it might be helpful to say something of their development.

3 Historical background and development

Of the subjects mentioned in the previous chapter *in vitro* fertilization, egg donation, embryo transfer and surrogacy are fairly recent
developments and for that reason only a little will be said about
their origins. By contrast artificial insemination has a much longer
history and this chapter is devoted almost entirely to an account of
its origins and development.

Although artificial insemination has been known for a considerable time the early accounts are of accidental, rather than deliberate,
insemination. Perhaps the first reference is to be found in the
Babylonian Talmud of the third century AD.[1] In the relevant
passage[2] a discussion takes place at a rabbinical academy in ancient
Palestine between the students and a distinguished Rabbi, Ben
Zoma, who lived in the second century AD. The subject is the
requirement that a high priest should marry a woman 'in her
virginity'.[3] The question which the students posed was whether a
woman who was pregnant, but was nevertheless *virgo intacta*, was
a fit person to marry a high priest. Ben Zoma said that there were
two possibilities. The first was that sexual intercourse had taken
place but by skilful manipulation of the penis the girl's hymen had
not been broken. While he regarded this as a remote possibility he
was of the opinion that because intercourse had taken place the
girl was not fit to marry a high priest. On the other hand, if the
pregnancy had occurred without sexual contact, the high priest
could marry the girl, and he pointed out that it was possible for a
woman to conceive as the result of bathing in water into which a
man had ejaculated.[4]

A second reference is to the conception of Ben Sira, who was
thought to be the son of the prophet Jeremiah. It was said that
some men, including Jeremiah, had ejaculated in a public bath.
Shortly afterwards his daughter came to bathe and she conceived
a child as the result of absorbing the semen released by her father.[5]

One further example is to be found in a work called *Hagakoth
S'mag* by Rabbi Peretz Ben Elijah of Corbeil in which he counselled

women against lying on bedsheets on which a man other than
their husbands had been lying. His point was that if the man had
deposited semen on the bedding and the woman became pregnant
as the result of coming in contact with it, the child might not know
the identity of his father and might, in ignorance, marry the father's
daughter. The Rabbi went on to say that a woman who had
conceived in this way was not guilty of adultery.[6]

In a case in Coblenz in 1905 a woman alleged that she had become
pregnant by scooping up some of her husband's semen from the
bedclothes and inserting it into her vagina. Despite medical
evidence that this was impossible the court accepted the woman's
account.[7]

Leaving aside these accounts of accidental impregnation, the earliest deliberate attempts at artificial insemination were with horses.
In the fourteenth century Arabs successfully impregnated well-
bred mares belonging to their enemies with semen from their own
poorer-quality stallions. They also used semen from their enemies'
superior stallions to impregnate their own inferior mares.[8]

There is some evidence that in the fifteenth century fish eggs
were artificially impregnated[9] but the first successful experiments
with fish are usually attributed to Ludwig Jacobi working in 1742.[10]
In 1780 an Italian professor, Spallanzani, successfully impregnated
a bitch by introducing semen into its uterus and some have
wondered why he did not apply the technique to humans.[11]

Artificial insemination in humans (AI)

There is some doubt about who was the first person to use human
artificial insemination. In 1550 Eustachius, a famous physician, was
consulted by a doctor's wife who was infertile. His advice was to
persuade her husband to insert his finger into her vagina after
intercourse and attempt to force the semen towards the mouth of
the uterus.[12] If we leave that account to one side, the first successful
human artificial insemination is usually credited to John Hunter, a
distinguished English physician of the eighteenth century. Hunter
may have performed the actual insemination or may simply have
given advice and it is not certain when this took place, as various
dates have been suggested.[13] However in 1799 an account of the
event was given to the Royal Society of London by Sir Everard
Home,[14] Hunter's brother-in-law, and he said that Hunter had done
his work prior to Spallanzani's experiments on dogs. Home's
description of the case is as follows:

A London cloth merchant suffering from hypospadias, which surgical intervention could not cure, entered into matrimony nevertheless. There was full emission during cohabitation, which proved that the testes were unimpaired, but the semen always escaped through the perineum. The late John Hunter was consulted in the hope of overcoming this disability and enabling the person in question to beget children. After various treatments had failed, Hunter proposed the following experiment: The husband was provided with a syringe, he was instructed to warm this and fill it with semen immediately after coitus, then injecting it into the vagina 'while the female organs were still under the influence of the coitus and in the proper state for receiving the semen'.

This was done and the woman gave birth, and neither Hunter nor the woman doubted this was the result of the experiment. This technique, using the semen from the husband (AIH), was repeated successfully by many others.

Schellen, the author of a major work on artificial insemination, observed that 'in none of the publications on AI up to 1900 is mention made of using semen from a donor; hence it must be supposed that all attempts were made with the husband's semen'.[15] It does not follow, however, that because none of the published work mentions the use of semen from a donor (AID) this technique was not used. The earliest account of its use appeared in *Medical World* in 1909 and described events which took place in 1884.[16] A. D. Hard, an American physician, reported that, while he was a student, he had assisted in the first successful AID. According to Hard the events took place in 1884 at the Samson Street Hospital of the Jefferson Medical College in Philadelphia. The experiment was carried out by a Professor Pancoast who had been consulted by a childless woman. Her husband admitted that as a young man he had contracted a mild form of gonorrhoea. The wife did not display any abnormality, and Pancoast concluded from an examination of the husband that the gonorrhoea had resulted in a blockage of the seminal ducts, which accounted for the absence of spermatozoa. At this point, according to Hard, one of the students remarked, seemingly as a joke, that the only solution was to use semen from another man. Whether as a result of this observation or not is unknown, but semen was collected from one of the students and it was introduced into the woman's uterus. At first neither the woman nor her husband was aware of the origin of the semen, but he was informed at a later stage. He was delighted that his wife was pregnant but decided that she should not be told about the method of conception. She later gave birth to a son whom Hard said resembled not the student but the husband. He also said that at the time of writing (1909) the son was in business in New York and that he had met him the previous year.

Hard's account produced a storm of protest.[17] One reader

concluded that he must have been dreaming, since Pancoast was a respectable man, and added: 'it is a gross crime to accuse Pancoast of "raping" the patient with semen "from the best-looking member of the class" '.[18] Another writer described AID as 'ethereal copulation'.[19] Hard replied to the effect that his account was based on fact, but he admitted that he deliberately added 'some personal comments with the object of setting men thinking'.[20]

However according to several authors AID was first used in the USA by Robert L. Dickinson, but they point out that his work was done in great secrecy.[21] Until the 1930s not much seems to have been written on the subject: one writer noted that by 1933 only twenty-four articles had appeared.[22]

Development in the USA

The first article of significance was published in 1941 in the *Journal of the American Medical Association*.[23] The authors were Seymour and Koerner, a husband and wife team who had sent questionnaires to 30 000 physicians practising in America, of whom only 7642 replied. Seymour and Koerner reported 9489 cases of women who had had at least one successful pregnancy by artificial insemination. Of these 5740 were the result of AIH and 3649 were from AID. Their overall success rate was 97 per cent but their results were the subject of trenchant criticism, not least because the success rate was very high.[24]

Further details about the practice in the United States can be seen in the Feversham Report of 1960. The evidence suggested that while there might have been isolated cases of AI during the latter part of the nineteenth century, AID was hardly practised at all until the 1920s. Eight practitioners advised the committee that they had had over 1000 pregnancies from AID up to 1959.[25]

More recently Curie-Cohen *et al.* published the results of investigations into the current practice of AID in the USA. They sent out 711 questionnaires to physicians who they thought were likely to be involved. They received 471 replies of which 379 said that they provided an AID service.[26]

Development in the UK

In the UK the first proper account appeared in 1945.[27] It listed 30 cases of AIH and 15 of AID. Of the cases of AIH 9 resulted in pregnancies and there were 4 live births. Of the 15 cases of AID there were 10 pregnancies and 8 live births. Fifteen years later, according to the Feversham Committee, AID was practised only on a very small scale and AIH had been 'carried out occasionally in at least 40 hospitals, but the witnesses said that "AIH is only rarely indicated as a suitable treatment" '.[28]

By 1971 the BMA had become aware of an increasing demand for information about AID and so they appointed a panel to inquire into the place of AID in our society. The BMA Panel requested assistance from 513 departments of obstetrics and gynaecology and received 315 replies. Of these 145 had been asked about AID but only 10 undertook the service. However more than 100 had referred patients to colleagues who were presumably in private practice.[29] The most recent survey was carried out by the RCOG in 1986. They received replies from 59 centres which were providing an AID service.[30]

Development in other countries

The Feversham Report contains some details about AI in other countries. This information was obtained from the Foreign Office, the Commonwealth Relations Office and the Colonial Office. The committee was also assisted by some published material and obtained advice from medical practitioners and others. It is not intended here to bring that information up to date in respect of all the eighteen countries mentioned in the Report. However developments in Australia and France will be mentioned, the first because recent data have been published, and the second because the French AID service is organized on a national basis.

Australia All that the Feversham Committee said about AI in Australia was that 'the practice of AIH is not uncommon . . . but AID is understood to be rare'.[31]This comment about AID is borne out by a report in the South African *Rand Daily Mail* in 1957 which was to the effect that AID had been 'entirely suspended in New South Wales, Victoria and Queensland, because of family breakdowns and the grave religious and legal problems created'.[32]

In a recent book, *Artificial Insemination by Donor*, J. F. Leeton traces the development of AID in Australia and observes that 'prior to 1970 there had been no medical report of any AID practice although it was carried out very infrequently by a few doctors in a clandestine manner'.[33] The first proper report, which appeared in 1970, described the treatment of 16 patients over a period of twenty-two years.[34] Professor Leeton concludes, 'It is evident that almost all the experience with AID in Australia began about 10 years ago and that most of the present-day work has originated within less than five years.'[35] However at the time of writing about 600 women were being treated with AID and he estimated that the demand might come from as many as 1000 women.[36]

France   According to Schellen,[37] after the experiment by Hunter it was not until 1865 that any publication on AI appeared. He continues, 'It is a striking fact that the renascence of AI took place chiefly in France'. A number of Frenchmen were involved in AIH in the second half of the nineteenth century but there seems to have been a decline later, with a revival on a small scale in the 1920s. The Feversham Committee noted that the subject had been discussed in France on a number of occasions, but that there was no legislation on the topic.[38]

In 1973 the practice of AID in France was systematized by the establishment of two sperm banks in Paris. In 1979 fifteen sperm banks had been established nationally, fourteen Centres for the Study and Preservation of Semen (CECOS), and the Centre of Human Functional Exploration (CEFER) which is situated in Marseille. The CECOS centres are located in university hospital centres but are not controlled by them. Instead they are managed by an administrative board which has representatives from the Ministry of Health, the hospital administration, the national health service and the medical profession. As far as the writer is aware that is the first and only AID service which operates on a national basis.[39]

Other countries   Clearly both AIH and AID are practised in other countries many of which were represented at the First International Symposium on Artificial Insemination and Semen Preservation held in Paris in 1979.[40] Among these are Belgium,[41] Switzerland,[42] Denmark,[43] Italy,[44] Spain,[45] Israel[46] and Canada.[47]

These observations about the development of AI have little impact or meaning unless one has some idea of how many children have been born as the result of this practice. Unfortunately it is not possible to give exact figures principally because those who have produced children as the result of artifical insemination, especially AID, usually do not wish to make this fact known. In the case of AIH children the register of births need not be annotated to show how the child was conceived; but even in a case where the child was conceived as the result of AID the register is unlikely to reveal that the husband was not the father.

More information might be available from medical practitioners, but they would probably regard the subject as confidential. Even if some did assist, it would not be possible to generalize from their involvement. Having sounded that cautionary note we shall now look at some of the figures which have been given and make some comment on how reliable they might be.

The earliest figures we have been able to trace for the USA were published in 1934. The author had interviewed about 200 physicians and concluded that 'some 50 to 150 babies may be born per year from artificial conception with donated sperm'.[48] The figures quoted by Seymour and Koerner in 1941 show the total number of conceptions, but the period during which these were achieved is not known. Ten years later Professor Ploscowe of New York University School of Law estimated that 20 000 children had been conceived as the result of AID.[49] In 1955 the *New York Post* suggested that the figure for the whole of the USA was 50 000 of which 10 000 were in New York City.[50] That figure of 50 000 was also given by *McCall's Magazine* in 1955, but it said that the annual birth rate was between 1000 and 1200.[51] As a result of their survey from 1977 to 1979 Curie-Cohen *et al.* thought that they could 'safely conclude that between 6000 and 10 000 children are born annually of this procedure'.[52] The advantage of the Curie-Cohen questionnaire is that it provides some basis for their figures whereas previous figures may be no more than guesswork, with varying degrees of inspiration.

Turning to the United Kingdom we find in a debate in the House of Lords in 1958 that widely-differing figures are given for the total number of children conceived as a result of AID. Dr Mary Barton who published the first report in the UK was quoted as estimating a total of 5000 children, but in the *News Chronicle* in February 1958 the figure given was 10 000, which was said to have been arrived at after consultation with eight medical practitioners. In the debate Lord Blackford suggested that the average of these two was probably accurate,[53] but Lord Amulree thought that the figure of 7000 was on the high side. He went on to say that he did not think that the figures involved would ever become very large or formidable.[54] Perhaps a more accurate estimate was given by the Feversham Committee in 1960 when it estimated an annual birth rate of 100 in the years preceding the Report.[55]

The BMA Panel did not give any indication of the number of children born as the result of AI, but the 1986 figure for AID conceptions known to the RCOG is 1442.

In vitro fertilization (IVF)

The first child to be conceived as the result of IVF was Louise Brown who was born in 1978. Her birth was the culmination of the combined efforts of Dr Robert Edwards, a physiologist, and Mr Patrick Steptoe, an obstetrician. Full details of this work over a ten-year period are recorded in their book, *A Matter of Life*, published in 1980. Dr Edwards's work began with animals and he later used his knowledge in that field in experiments with human sperm and eggs.[56] Shortly after the birth of Louise Brown, Edwards and Steptoe set up a private IVF clinic at Bourn Hall near Cambridge. Since its opening over 200 children have been born including twins and

triplets. IVF is also practised on the NHS and there are a number
of centres including those in London, Glasgow and Aberdeen. IVF
is also undertaken in other countries but mainly in the USA and
Australia.

Conception by IVF involves the fertilization of an ovum *in vitro*
(in a glass) and the resulting embryo is replaced in the woman's
uterus. At one time this replacement process was described by
some as 'embryo transfer', but more recently the term 'embryo
transfer' has been used to describe the implantation of the embryo
in another woman.

Egg donation

This occurs where a woman donates an egg or eggs to another. It
has been attempted in the USA and in Australia where there has
been at least one live birth.[57]

Embryo transfer (or donation)

As early as 1973 Dr Edwards commented that it was easier to
transfer an embryo to another woman; but it was not until 1983
that scientists published details of their efforts to produce a child
from a donated embryo,[58] and early in 1984 the first child was born
in Australia as the result of embryo donation.[59] It is perhaps too
early to say what further developments there will be in this area.
Embryo donation is however a reality.

Surrogacy

As we shall see later the terminology in this area is confused. What
is usually meant by the term 'surrogacy' is that one woman agrees
to conceive and carry a child for another. Unlike most of the other
procedures considered in this book surrogacy does not necessarily
require the involvement of the medical profession. It may therefore
have gone on for centuries. Indeed some people cite the biblical
experience of Abraham as the first example of surrogacy. Genesis
16 discloses that Abraham's wife Sarah was infertile and she asked
the Lord to ensure that Abraham would be able to father a child
by Sarah's maidservant Hagar, and subsequently a son, Ishmael,
was born.

Whether or not surrogacy is a practice of some antiquity may be
open to doubt, but what is clear is that in the last few years it
has received considerable publicity, especially in America where
agencies have been set up to make surrogacy arrangements.[60]

A detailed consideration of the various legal, ethical and social issues created by surrogacy has not yet taken place, principally because it is only in these recent years that much attention has focused on it.

Having given a brief sketch of these various techniques, we shall now look at their practice and the issues this raised.

PART II
ARTIFICIAL
INSEMINATION

4 Artificial insemination

As will be obvious from the discussion in the following chapters, AIH creates fewer legal problems than AID, but as a background for the discussion of the legal issues which arise from both practices, it is appropriate to mention briefly the circumstances in which each would be used.

AIH

It is misleading to use the term 'AIH' when the semen which is used is that of the male partner of a couple who are not married. What one can say however is that the circumstances which are appropriate for the use of AIH would also be appropriate for using the semen from the male partner of a cohabiting couple. In that connection, but only there, 'AIH' is used to cover both the use of a husband's semen and that of a male partner where the couple are not married.

Indications for AIH[1]

There are two main reasons why AIH is used. One is where it is difficult or impossible for the male to deposit semen into the vagina; the other is where the male is infertile.

An inability to deposit semen into the vagina may have a number of causes. For example there may be an abnormality in the penis or the male may be impotent. He may suffer from retrograde ejaculation, which means that the semen collects in the bladder and is not expelled externally. Alternatively the woman's cervical fluid may be hostile to the semen and so prevents or impedes its passage to the neck of the womb. In addition obesity, vaginal tumours or constriction of the vagina may make intercourse difficult or impossible.

The second indication is infertility. The semen may be defective because it contains few sperm, or the volume of the ejaculate is low, or the sperm which are produced do not move as freely as they should for fertilization to take place. Not surprisingly the use of AIH in these circumstances has in general yielded poor results.[2] That being so, it is likely that the couple would be advised to undergo AID.

Indications for AID

AID will be appropriate principally where the problem is sperm deficiency.[3] The seminal fluid may not contain any sperm, or the sperm may be dead, or the male may appear to be sub-fertile. In some cases a woman may develop antibodies to her husband's semen and so AID would be indicated.

It may be that the male is fertile but he suffers, or may suffer, from some disorder which could be transmitted to his children. conditions such as Klinefelter's Syndrome (the XYY man), which is a chromosomal defect, or some hereditary or familial disease such as cysticfibrosis could be passed on to his children. If there is such a risk AID could eliminate it. AID could also be used where there is severe Rhesus incompatibility between the man and the woman.

While, as we have said, the success rate for AIH is low, that for AID is much higher, but the literature discloses success rates which vary enormously, from as low as 37 per cent[4] to as high as 84 per cent.[5] The most common figures are between 60 and 70 per cent.[6]

In Chapter 5 the legal issues arising from the use of AIH will be examined and then in the three following chapters, those arising from the use of AID.

5 AIH

AIH is no more than assisted fertilization and it does not involve anyone other than the couple and probably a medical practitioner. No extraneous element is introduced into the couple's relationship and perhaps for that reason it gives rise to fewer legal problems than AID. Nevertheless the issues it does raise are complex and important. The principal issue is the effect which it has on a marriage, but there are a number of other points which can be dealt with briefly.

Consent

Before embarking on AIH the medical practitioner should obtain the necessary consent. If he fails to obtain consent from the man or the woman for any physical examination, or the woman's consent for the insemination, he would technically commit an assault. It is highly unlikely that a doctor would proceed in this way and so the issue does not merit further comment.

Degree of skill

In addition to obtaining the consent of the patient(s) the doctor must exercise the degree of skill which would be expected of a reasonably competent member of his profession. If he fails to do so and as a result injures his patient, he would be liable for damages. Again, a claim of this nature is unlikely to arise in connection with AIH, but it is possible, though improbable, that the doctor may injure the patient during the physical examination or while performing the insemination. A claim for damages is more likely to arise out of a doctor's involvement with AID, and these issues are explored more fully later.

Effect on marriage

By far the most important issue is the effect of AIH on the marriage. (What follows clearly relates only to a married couple, since AI has no legal effect on the relationship between cohabiting couples.) There are three points. The first is whether a marriage is consummated if the woman undergoes AIH. The second is whether AIH would prevent either party from setting aside (annulling) a marriage which could otherwise be annulled (approbation or homologation); and the third is whether AIH would amount to condonation of a matrimonial offence, in particular adultery. The first two topics also raise the question of the status of a child born as the result of AIH, which in turn has a bearing on issues such as maintenance, custody and succession.

AIH and consummation

In Scotland, England and many of the American states, a marriage may be annulled if either of the parties is impotent.[1] For this purpose 'impotence' is a permanent and incurable inability to have sexual intercourse with the other spouse and, in Scotland but not in England, the defect must have existed at the time the marriage was entered into.[2] The reason for the rule is that since the time of the Canon Law (pre-Reformation) marriage has been regarded as a contract, one of the implied conditions being that each of the parties could consummate it. In England,[3] and also in some states in the USA,[4] wilful refusal to consummate a marriage is also a ground for setting the marriage aside, but this is not so in Scotland.[5] In some jurisdictions the difference between annulling a marriage and divorce is that a marriage which is annulled is regarded for most purposes as never having existed, whereas a valid marriage terminated by divorce subsists until the divorce takes place.

It is important to draw a distinction between infertility and impotence. A man who is infertile may be perfectly capable of having sexual intercourse. He is not impotent, but will not be able to father children. By contrast a man who is impotent may be fertile and could father children, but his wife may have to be artificially inseminated because of his inability to have sexual intercourse. A woman may also be impotent if she is unable to have sexual intercourse.

The issue which arises is whether artificial insemination is equivalent to 'sexual intercourse'. Before that can be answered it is necessary to consider the legal meaning of sexual intercourse. In Scotland there has been very little discussion on this point, but recently it has been held that it means full and complete intercourse in the ordinary sense of the word,[6] a view shared by the leading textbook writer.[7]

By contrast in England there has been a great deal of case law, not in relation to impotence but in connection with wilful non-consummation. The distinguished nineteenth-century judge Dr Lushington said: 'Sexual intercourse, in the proper meaning of the term, is ordinary and complete intercourse; it does not mean partial or imperfect intercourse.'[8] Of itself, that observation does not take matters much further, but Dr Lushington's comment has been more fully explained in relation to two practices; one is condomistic intercourse and the other is *coitus interruptus*.

In a case in 1948 a husband petitioned the court to annul his marriage on the ground that his wife refused to have intercourse unless he used a contraceptive sheath. The husband argued that the marriage had not been consummated. However the House of Lords held that condomistic intercourse did not prevent the intercourse from being 'ordinary and complete' and that the marriage had been consummated.[9] Accordingly all that would appear to be required for consummation of a marriage is penetration of the female by the male, and it would seem to follow that the practice of *coitus interruptus* would not prevent a marriage from being consummated. The House of Lords did not express an opinion on this point and subsequent case law is divided on the matter.[10] However the better view would seem to be that penetration is both necessary and sufficient for consummation.[11]

The position in the USA is similar. One leading compendium of US law, the *Corpus Iuris Secundum*, contains the following comment:

A marriage of one physically incapable of sexual intercourse has been held to be invalid. Physical incapacity consists in an incapacity for true and natural copulation or 'copula vera', partial, imperfect or unnatural copula not being within the definition.[12]

That is illustrated by a case in New Jersey. In *T. v. M*,[13] a husband petitioned for annulment of the marriage on the ground that his wife was impotent. The wife was medically examined and was found to be a virgin. Nevertheless she had had a miscarriage. There was medical evidence that this was a 'splash pregnancy' caused by the husband ejaculating against his wife's vulva while attempting to have normal sexual intercourse. The court declared the marriage to be null.

Most states have statutory provisions which enable a marriage to be annulled on the ground of incurable impotence.[14] The Uniform Marriage and Divorce Act has a similar provision under which a court may declare a marriage invalid, 'if a party lacks physical capacity to consummate the marriage by sexual intercourse, and at the time the marriage was solemnized the other party did not know of the incapacity'.[15] The law in South Africa,[16] Canada[17] and Australia[18] is similar. It is against that background that we return to the question whether AIH can be regarded as 'sexual intercourse'.

This point has not arisen for decision in any reported case, but the opinion of textbook writers is that artificial insemination, even using the husband's semen, does not constitute sexual intercourse because it does not involve penetration. Support for that view can be had from cases involving fecundation *ab extra*. One example is *Clarke v. Clarke*[19] where the medical evidence was inconclusive on the question whether the marriage had been consummated, but the husband admitted that the wife had given birth to a child of which he was the father. The court accepted his evidence that the wife had been impregnated *ab extra* and that the marriage had never been consummated. Accordingly decree of nullity was granted.

Further support comes from the decision of Lord Wheatley in the Scottish case of *MacLennan v. MacLennan*[20] which raised the question whether a woman who undergoes AID without her husband's consent has committed adultery. Although this case is not directly in point, Lord Wheatley held that for adultery to take place the parties had to have sexual intercourse.[21] In that connection he said:

> The placing of the male seed in the female ovum [*sic*] need not necessarily result from the sexual act, and if it does not, but is placed there by some other means, there is no sexual intercourse.[22]

A husband's impotence or wilful refusal to consummate a marriage could therefore still permit a wife to have the marriage set aside on the ground that her husband was unable or unwilling to have sexual intercourse and it would not be a defence to show that she had been artificially inseminated by him, or by a donor.

AIH as homologation or approbation

However the remedy we have just discussed may not be available if the wife has acted in such a way that it can be assumed that she is prepared to overlook the defect. What is important in this context is the wife's conduct. If the wife knows about the existence of a remedy but acts in such a way as to indicate that she does not regard the marriage as imperfect, then she will be prevented from founding on the impotence or wilful refusal in any action of annulment of the marriage. In Scotland this conduct is known as homologation,[23] but in the Anglo-American jurisdictions a variety of terms are used: approbation, ratification, acquiescence, estoppel.[24]

The issue is whether the fact that a wife undergoes AIH can amount to homologation or approbation, but it remains unsettled in English law despite having been discussed in two cases.[25] It has also been debated by a Commission appointed by the Archbishops of Canterbury and York, which reported in 1955;[26] by the Royal Commission on Marriage and Divorce in 1956;[27] the Feversham Committee in 1960;[28] and the (English) Law Commission in 1968.[29]

In the first of the two cases, *REL v. EL*[30] the wife had undergone AIH and became pregnant. Some time later the parties stopped living together, but the wife gave birth to a child some eight months thereafter. She raised an action to have the marriage annulled on the ground of her husband's inability or wilful refusal to have sexual intercourse. However it was clear from her evidence that the principal reason why she had undergone AIH was to conceive a child, in the hope that its birth would enable her and her husband to have normal sexual relations. It was held that the marriage had not been approbated because the husband was not under the impression that his wife had in any way accepted their abnormal marriage.

In the subsequent case of *Slater v. Slater*[31] the wife had AID but she failed to conceive. The parties then adopted a child, but both the AID and the adoption took place before the wife was made aware that she had grounds for having the marriage annulled. Accordingly the court held that the marriage had not been approbated. A similar decision was reached in *Q v. Q*,[32] where the court referred to the recommendations of the Royal Commission on Marriage and Divorce, which are discussed below, but pointed out that these had not yet become law and since the wife had been unaware of her legal remedy of annulment when she had undergone AID there was no approbation, and the marriage was annulled.

The Commission appointed by the Archbishops thought that artificial insemination should amount to approbation of a marriage only if 'a child has resulted from the joint act, or with consent of both parties', but that the birth of such a child however conceived should be regarded as approbation.[33] By contrast the Royal Commission thought that where the wife had had AIH or AID, that should be regarded as approbation.[34] The Feversham Committee recommended that 'the fact that a live child has been born as a result of artificial insemination of a woman with the seed of her husband should be a bar to proceedings for nullity of marriage on the ground of impotence'[35] and they made a similar recommendation about AID.[36] These differing views were considered by the Law Commission in their Working Paper[37] and they requested comments on this topic.[38] These were likewise divided and so the Law Commission did not recommend any change in the law. The Nullity of Marriage Act 1971 which implements the Royal

Commission's Report does not mention artificial insemination, and the question still remains open whether AIH and AID can amount to approbation.

The position in Scotland is also uncertain, the only authority being the case of *AB v. CB*[39] where the wife's physical condition (a tight band in the lower vagina) prevented her from having normal sexual relations. However she was given AIH and subsequently gave birth to a child, which the couple adopted. Some six years later they adopted a second child. The court took the view that these acts amounted to homologation, but it is not entirely clear from the judgment whether the artificial insemination was regarded in itself as sufficient, although it seems that it may have been. Lord Walker said:

> . . . what is to be said of the act of the parties in giving and receiving artificial insemination? It seems to me out of the question to suppose that they could have agreed to do what they did than except on the footing that they intended to treat their imperfect marriage as if it were perfect. But assuming that the insemination could be regarded as being a homologation conditional upon a child being born – of which there is no evidence – their act did not stand alone because it was followed by the birth of a child. I think that the parties must have intended that the child should be regarded as the child of a marriage no longer imperfect and voidable, but valid and binding.
>
> But the matter does not rest on that incident alone, because after a lapse of some six years, when both parties must have been perfectly aware that their marriage was incapable of consummation, they both agreed to adopt and did adopt a second child. That action seems to me to be an overt fact which yields and can only yield, the inference that the husband and wife intended to treat their imperfect marriage as a perfect and valid one.[40]

It seems to have been his lordship's opinion that the consent to, and obtaining of, AIH amounted to homologation. That was the view of the Royal Commission on Marriage and Divorce and it is submitted that this is the correct approach. What is important is the attitude of the parties, in particular that of the wife who may be able to petition the court to have the marriage set aside. Her knowledge and conduct in the light of that knowledge matters more than the result of her actions. Once the woman has been artificially inseminated she has no control over whether she becomes pregnant nor whether the pregnancy will have a successful outcome. Therefore the emphasis should be placed on her consent and the fact that she has been artificially inseminated, and not on whether she conceived or gave birth. It is to be hoped that this view will find favour with any legislature which is contemplating acting on the matter.

In South African law the issues have not been resolved, but the leading writer is of the opinion that where a wife undergoes AIH or AID with her husband's consent that will usually amount to approbation.[41] However he sounded a cautionary note by reference to the English cases of *REL v. EL* and *Slater v. Slater*. In Australia a petitioner will be barred from annulling a marriage because of her conduct, which it is noted is characterized as 'approbation'.[42]

Writing of the position in Canada, Mendes da Costa says:

> The test of approbation [acquiescence, ratification] is whether the petitioner, with full knowledge of the respondent's incurable incapacity and the legal rights and remedies arising therefrom, had 'affirmatively accepted and contentedly acquiesced' in the marriage. Where the wife has, with her husband's concurrence, undergone artificial insemination, or the spouses have jointly adopted a child, she will normally have been considered to have acquiesced in her husband's impotence . . .

but this writer also says that everything depends on the circumstances and refers to the two English cases.[43]

In the USA the law recognizes that one spouse may by his or her conduct be barred from setting aside a marriage. A general statement of this doctrine is to be found in a recent case in the Supreme Court of Pennsylvania, where it was said:

> In a suit for nullity of a marriage, where, as here, the facts and circumstances so plainly imply that the complaining spouse recognised the existence and validity of the marriage and accepted the status of husband and wife, it would be most inequitable and contrary to public policy that he or she should be permitted to treat the marriage relation as if it had never existed.[44]

However, although that general statement might be applied to a wife who has had AID with her husband's consent, it was not argued in any of the American cases. In *Gursky v. Gursky*,[45] for example, the marriage was set aside on the ground of the husband's impotence, but the fact that he had consented to her having AID prevented him from refusing to maintain the child.

Although the position remains uncertain the writers all emphasize the need to ascertain whether the woman knew of her remedy and the reason why she agreed to undergo artificial insemination. The matter does not arise very often, but if the mere fact that a woman undergoes AI is to be regarded as homologation or approbation, that shifts the emphasis away from knowledge and intention and would have wider implications than cases of AI.

AIH as condonation

The third issue arises where a wife's conduct has been such that
it provides the husband with grounds for divorce, but she later
undergoes artificial insemination. The point is whether that would
bar her husband from founding on such conduct in an action for
divorce – in other words whether the husband had condoned his
wife's conduct.

In England prior to 1969, and in Scotland prior to 1976, divorce
law was based on the theory of the matrimonial offence. This meant
that, although in the opinion of the parties and their associates the
marriage was at an end, and even though the parties wished to be
free of each other, a divorce could not be granted unless a matrimonial offence had been committed. Matrimonial offences include
cruelty, desertion and adultery.

However a divorce would not be granted if the offence had been
condoned. In layman's terms condonation means forgiveness, but
in law the spouse who had committed the offence had to be
reinstated in his or her former position in the household, that
is, the parties must have resumed cohabitation. Furthermore the
reinstatement had to be made in the knowledge of all the material
facts and with the intention of not enforcing the rights which had
accrued as the result of the conduct. What amounted to a resumption of cohabitation was a question of fact. In Scotland sexual intercourse is probably neither necessary nor conclusive of condonation,[46] but in England one act of intercourse would amount to
condonation.[47]

When the Feversham Committee considered whether AIH could
be regarded as condonation, they thought that: 'the court's decision
might well turn on whether or not the insemination had resulted
in the birth of a child'.[48] This reflects their view on approbation but
it is difficult to see why this should be so. In Scotland at least, a
matrimonial offence can be condoned even though the parties do
not have intercourse, and even if they do, that is not conclusive.
It follows therefore that the birth of a child is neither necessary nor
conclusive. In England, while one act of intercourse would amount
to condonation, it would not necessarily result in the birth of a
child. Nevertheless the committee suggested that in the case where
a wife undergoes artificial insemination the birth of the child is of
importance.

What is significant in determining whether a matrimonial offence
has been condoned is the same as in homologation, namely the
attitude of the parties to each other. While it could be argued that
by consenting to the artificial insemination the husband has
forgiven his wife, in Scotland it is necessary to ascertain whether

she has been reinstated to her former position in the household. If she has not, then there can be no condonation. In England, because one act of sexual intercourse amounts to condonation, the question is whether artificial insemination is 'sexual intercourse'. As noted earlier, it is not, and hence it will not amount to condonation.

The reforms in the divorce laws in 1969[49] and 1976[50] intended to remove the notion of the matrimonial offence and replace it with a single ground of divorce, namely that the marriage has irretrievably broken down. However a court will not hold that the marriage has irretrievably broken down unless at least one of five 'facts' is proved. These include what might loosely be termed 'intolerable conduct', desertion and adultery.[51] Under the English provisions the traditional concept of condonation in relation to divorce was removed, but in Scotland it remains a defence to an action based on adultery.[52]

However in both countries attempts at reconciliation are encouraged and the Acts contain provisions which enable the parties to resume living together for a limited period without adversely affecting their rights to a divorce. In both England and Scotland the period is six months.[53]

The question which arises is what significance, if any, can be attached to the fact that during the period permitted by the legislation for reconciliation the wife undergoes artificial insemination with her husband's consent.

The phrase 'lived together' which appears in the English statute is not defined[54] but it would be equivalent to the Scottish term 'cohabit'[55] which is defined in the Act: '[T]he parties to a marriage shall be held to cohabit with one another only when they are in fact living together as man and wife.'[56] While one can say that sexual intercourse is a normal part of married life, its absence does not demonstrate that the parties have not resumed cohabitation nor does its presence demonstrate that they have. It is submitted that the court would take a similar approach where the wife has undergone artificial insemination. Accordingly the fact that the wife has been artificially inseminated will not of itself amount to a resumption of cohabitation.

In South Africa the position is that the spouse must not only be forgiven but must also be restored to his/her former position.[57] Verbal forgiveness without resumption of cohabitation and restoration of all marital rights does not amount to condonation. One leading South African judge said that condonation:

> means something more than mere pardon or forgiveness which might conceivably be accorded by the injured spouse as a matter of Christian duty without any idea of restoring the *status quo ante* . . . Forgiveness

by the injured spouse of the infidelity of his or her partner, if it is to operate as a bar to subsequent proceedings founded on the offence, must contemplate the restoration of the offending spouse to his or her previous position, and must result in a reconciliation between the two. The injured spouse must have knowledge of the offence, must fully forgive it, and must be prepared to take back the guilty party, the latter must be willing to accept the forgiveness and to take advantage of the pardon, and a reconciliation must ensue.[58]

In that connection, one textbook writer observes that sexual intercourse in the full knowledge of the other spouse's adultery is, normally, conclusive evidence of condonation.[59] The positions in Australia[60] and Canada[61] largely mirror English law.

The result is a sensible one. In the various jurisdictions which have been looked at the approach has not been to look at the artificial insemination in isolation. It is important to examine the conduct of the parties, particularly the husband, and attempt to ascertain whether the wife has been forgiven and restored to the position she had before the act of adultery. In reaching a decision the artificial insemination can be only one factor. If, for example, a husband was fertile and potent but his wife had had AI, that would be viewed in a different light from AI undertaken where the husband was impotent or infertile.

Status of children born as the result of AIH

When a woman gives birth to a child as the result of AIH there is no doubt that her husband is the father of the child and so the child will be legitimate. However a marriage which is voidable might be set aside by the courts and it would then be regarded in law for many purposes as if it had never existed. Thus in the United Kingdom before the position was altered by statute, if a child had been born as the result of AIH into a marriage which was voidable and was later annulled, the child would be illegitimate. In *REL v. EL*[62] the court declared the child to be illegitimate, but the judge said that was 'most regrettable' and the position was altered by the Law Reform (Miscellaneous Provisions) Act 1949. The Act applies in Scotland and England and provides that where a decree of nullity is granted in respect of a voidable marriage, a child of that marriage shall be deemed to be the legitimate child of the parties if it would have been legitimate in the event of the marriage being dissolved by divorce or death.[63] Accordingly, because a child born as the result of AIH would be legitimate if a couple are divorced, it would be legitimate if the marriage is annulled.

In the United States most states have similar statutory

provisions.[64] As one would expect however, there are considerable variations between states. Some statutory provisions cover void and voidable marriages, while some others except incestuous, bigamous and miscegenetic marriages. The statutes which make children legitimate even though they are born into void or voidable marriages have received a liberal interpretation. They have been used to declare an AID child legitimate, even though such children were not specifically covered by the provisions. They have also been interpreted in favour of legitimizing children born into a common law marriage in a state which did not recognize such marriages. In the light of such liberal policy it seems unlikely that a court would hold a child born as the result of AIH to be illegitimate.

Succession and maintenance

If by statutory provision or court decision AIH children are legitimate, they will have the same rights of succession and maintenance as other legitimate children. If on the other hand the children are illegitimate, it would depend on the legal system what rights, if any, they have against their parents' estate. Some states treat legitimate and illegitimate children in the same way; in others the distinctions are marked; and in others the policy is to minimize the distinction. In others still, the concept of 'illegitimacy' does not exist. That variety of approaches would require a detailed analysis and explanation which would be out of place in a book such as this.

Conclusion

AIH can give rise to interesting and complex legal issues. Those discussed above are the main ones but they have not arisen very often and they might not be regarded by a couple contemplating AIH as very important. However they would want to know whether the law regarded the child as legitimate (or the equivalent). A decision on that point could turn on some of the other matters just raised.

One variant of AIH which clearly could give rise to considerable legal difficulties is where it is used after the husband's death. This is dealt with later.[65]

6 AID as a ground of divorce

For some time, much of the legal discussion of AID focused on the question whether it gave a husband grounds for divorce. Where the insemination had been done without his consent, 'non-consensual AID', the issue was whether AID amounts to adultery. In many jurisdictions divorce is available only on specified grounds. Accordingly before a divorce would be granted a party would have to establish one or other of these grounds. If he failed divorce would not be granted, even though the marriage was truly at an end. The reason why adultery should be chosen is not difficult to see. When children are born as the result of AID the husband is not the father. The clearest analogy is of a child born as the result of an adultery; hence the attempt to equate AID, particularly non-consensual AID, with adultery. A further issue however is, if AID is not adultery would it permit a divorce on some other ground?

AID as adultery

There are three main approaches to this matter. The first is to examine definitions of adultery in statutes, reported cases and other sources, for example dictionaries. The second approach involves looking at the grounds of divorce (which are usually laid down by statute) in a particular jurisdiction and attempting to ascertain their underlying purpose. The third is a multidisciplinary approach, consisting of an examination of present attitudes – medical, ethical, sociological and psychological – towards the practice of AID with a view to formulating a policy which would clarify the divorce issue.

Definitions

Before considering any definitions it should be noted that they may have been framed before AID was practised on any significant scale.

Accordingly there can be no certainty that a definition framed with AID in mind would take the same form.

The *Oxford English Dictionary* defines 'adultery' as 'violation of the marriage bed: the voluntary sexual intercourse of a married person with one of the opposite sex, whether unmarried, or married to another'. It has been said that the term 'adultery' has no special meaning in law, and one English judge, Karminski J., observed: 'Nobody has yet attempted to define adultery, and I do not propose to rush in where wiser men have not.'[1] Despite that observation, there are definitions in various jurisdictions and these bear a marked resemblance to the one in the *Oxford English Dictionary*. For example, the Californian Civil Code defines adultery as 'the voluntary sexual intercourse of a married person with a person other than the offender's husband or wife'.[2] A similar approach can be seen in definitions in other statutes, in reported cases and legal dictionaries.

Although these definitions may appear to be relatively simple and leave little or no room for doubt as to what adultery involves, it is not simplistic to consider what is meant by the phrase 'sexual intercourse'. In popular parlance, it means some physical contact between male and female sexual organs and, on that basis, it is difficult to see how a court could equate AID (even without the husband's consent) with adultery. In AID the semen is transmitted mechanically and without the presence of the donor; indeed physicians try to ensure that the identities of the donor and recipient are never revealed to each other. Given the separation of the act of producing the semen from the insemination itself, there is no sexual gratification nor emotional involvement such as is usually associated with adultery. For these reasons the donor cannot be regarded as having committed adultery with the recipient.

As an alternative it might be suggested that the doctor is to be regarded as committing adultery. However he does not provide the semen, the emotional element again is absent and given that the person who performs the insemination might be female, it seems improbable that a court would take the view that the doctor had committed adultery.

On the other hand, since a legal concept can be adapted to meet the needs of a new situation, one could argue that because AID involves the reproductive organs of both the donor and recipient, semen is transmitted and pregnancy may result, in those respects it is identical with adultery. It could therefore be suggested that it is adultery, because both involve the surrender of the reproductive organs outside marriage. Some support for that view may be had from a statement by a distinguished United Kingdom judge, Lord Dunedin, in the case of *Russell v. Russell*[3] where he said, 'fecundation *ab extra* is, I doubt not, adultery'. While that statement is undoubtedly of high authority and can be regarded as extending the definitions of adultery mentioned above, it was made without AID in mind and, accordingly, less weight should be attached to it than a statement about adultery which was made in a case involving AID. In that connection it is appropriate to examine the case of *Orford v.Orford*,[4] the first reported case on artificial insemination. In the Supreme Court of Ontario, Orde J. described AID as 'a monstrous act of adultery' because it involved 'the voluntary surrender to another person of the reproductive powers or faculties of the guilty person; and any submission of these powers to the services or enjoyment of any person other than the husband or wife comes within the definition of "adultery" '.

Several points can be made about that statement. In the first place it was not strictly necessary for the decision of the case (in legal parlance it was *obiter*). The husband had asserted that his wife had committed adultery by undergoing AID without his consent, but the court found that the wife had committed adultery in the ordinary way. Accordingly it was not necessary to say anything about AID. Furthermore the use of the phrase 'guilty person' seems to beg the question.

Of more importance is the use of the phrase 'reproductive powers or faculties'. This would logically cover a woman who undergoes a gynaecological examination, or the husband who submits to a urological examination or seminal analysis. In these circumstances there is a submission of the 'reproductive powers or faculties' to a person who is not the other spouse. It would seem absurd, however, to equate such conduct with adultery. Given the emphasis on 'reproductive powers or faculties', it would follow that anyone who does not have these, for example post-menopausal women and persons who are sterile, would not come into this category, and cannot be guilty of adultery.

Although that suggestion might also seem bizarre, it is supported by a later statement in the judgment, where the judge observed that the essence of adultery lay not in any 'moral turpitude' or in the physical contact, but rather in the fact that 'in the case of the woman, it involves the possibility of introducing into the family of the husband a false strain of blood. Any act on the part of the wife which does that, would, therefore be adulterous'. If there was no risk of a 'false strain of blood', there would presumably be no adultery. Another point is that the mention of the possibility of the wife having illegitimate children suggests that it might be necessary to produce a different definition of adultery to deal with a husband's conduct.

Since the decision in *Orford v. Orford* there have been a number of other cases in which a different approach has been taken.[5] That in itself casts some doubt on the validity of Orde's view, but the fact that there are other views does not of itself make his wrong. However, as has been suggested, his definition of adultery is wide enough to cover other activities which would not be regarded as adultery, while other conduct which would commonly be thought of as adultery would not come within Orde's definition.

However, 'dictionary' type definitions of 'adultery' are not particularly helpful. Those which have been noted contain phrases which themselves require explanation, and it might therefore be preferable to examine the background to divorce legislation to ascertain whether conduct which would be grounds for divorce would include a wife undergoing AID. This approach would be especially appropriate where the jurisdiction did not have a definition of adultery.

Reasons why adultery provides a ground for divorce

Any attempt to ascertain why adultery is a ground of divorce must obviously examine the history of the legislative provisions. It is not possible to examine a large number of jurisdictions, and so a few of significance have been selected.

Scotland   Divorce was introduced in Scotland in 1563[6] shortly after the Reformation. The relevant Act, although permitting divorce on the ground of adultery, does not give a definition of adultery and merely describes it as 'a filthy vice and crime'. Given that the Reformers based their views (albeit somewhat unconvincingly) upon two biblical passages,[7] they probably considered that it was unnecessary to give reasons for making it a ground for divorce. One Scottish judge observed:[8]

> Some of our great legal writers . . . do not even seek to define it [adultery], while others, in referring to it, use terms which are more descriptive than definitive. This may be due to the fact that in earlier days, when life was regulated by the natural rather than the scientific order of things, people knew what was meant by adultery and what its concomitants were.

Two of the principal legal writers in Scotland mentioned by the judge, namely Stair and Erskine, do not define adultery, far less give reasons why it was a ground for divorce. However, one early nineteenth-century writer, Baron David Hume, stated:[9]

> The second obligation of the married pair is that of fidelity to the marriage bed . . . This, though certainly true of both parties, is more especially so on the part of the female, whose infidelity extinguishes all

affection to the husband, may impose a spurious offspring on him, and is utterly destructive to the welfare of the house and family, and has therefore in all countries, and even in the earliest stages of society, been considered as a crime in some measure and a fit object of public animadversion.

England In England after the Reformation the doctrine of indissolubility of marriage prevailed and the ecclesiastical courts, which had jurisdiction over such matters, could not grant a decree of divorce which would permit the parties to remarry (divorce *a vinculo matrimonii*). Prior to 1857 the only method of obtaining such a divorce was a private Act of Parliament, which was costly.[10] However recommendations of the commission appointed to investigate divorce[11] led to the Matrimonial Causes Act 1857, which permitted divorce *a vinculo matrimonii* on the ground of adultery. The commission regarded adultery as:

> an offence which destroys altogether the primary objects of the married state, by in some instances a confusion of offspring; by cutting off, in others, all hope of succession; by diverting in all the affection and feelings into strange channels, which reason and religion forbade them to flow in.[12]

USA The American colonies did not have the ecclesiastical courts which had jurisdiction over divorce in England,[13] but some, for example those in the South, adhered fairly strictly to the English pattern by adopting the ecclesiastical rules about marriage and divorce.[14] Others such as the western states permitted divorce on fairly wide grounds, including desertion and adultery.[15] These different approaches are still reflected in the present divorce laws.[16] One common ground for divorce is adultery, but the reason for its existence as a ground is not clear.[17] Nevertheless in a divorce action at the beginning of the present century the notion of confusion of offspring was mentioned as being the reason for permitting divorce on that ground. In *State v. Roberts*[18] it was said: 'Adultery was condemned because it tended to introduce spurious heirs into a family and to adulterate the issue of an innocent husband and turn the inheritance away from his own blood to that of a stranger.'

Non-legal comments

There are of course other writings on this topic and the following are noteworthy. Dr Samuel Johnson was of the view that 'confusion of progeny constitutes the essence of the crime' of adultery.[19] Bertrand Russell in *Marriage and Morals* states[20] that 'adultery in itself, should not . . . be a ground of divorce' but continues: 'In

saying this I am, of course, assuming that the adulterous union
will not be such as to lead to children. Where illegitimate children
come in, the issue is much more complicated . . . This goes against
the biological basis of marriage.'

Other reasons have been given for condemning adultery. It has
been said that adultery 'involves violation of a spouse's right to
sexual exclusivity in his mate',[21] and that view would have the
support of at least one anthropologist: in *The History of Human
Marriage*, Westermarck[22] gives as the main reason for the opposition
to adultery in primitive societies that this loss which the husband
suffers gives rise to feelings of jealousy with which society would
sympathize. That point is developed in his *Origin and Development
of the Moral Ideas*[23] where he describes the extreme severity with
which adultery was treated, and continues:

> In early civilisation the husband has often extreme rights over his wife.
> The seducer encroaches upon a right of which he is most jealous, and
> with regard to which his passions are most easily inflamed. Adultery is
> regarded as an illegitimate appropriation of the exclusive claims which
> the husband has acquired by the purchase of his wife, as an offence
> against property . . . Modern legislation . . . does not to the same extent
> as early law and custom allow a man to give free bent to his angry
> passion; it regards the dishonour of the aggrieved husband as a matter
> of too private a nature to be publicly avenged; and the faithfulness
> which a wife owes her husband is no longer connected with any idea
> of ownership.

Putting these various theories together, one could suggest that
adultery by the wife was condemned because it amounted to an
invasion of the husband's proprietorial rights in his wife, or that it
gave rise to feelings of jealousy and perhaps also fear of alienation
of affection and that the husband suffered social stigma as a result.
Adultery might also be condemned because of the risk of introducing an illegitimate child into the family, which might in turn
give rise to concern about its stability.[24]

Theories about adultery and the practice of AID

Having mentioned some of the theories behind permitting divorce
on the grounds of adultery, we must now consider the extent to
which these theories can accommodate the practice of AID.

The first reason given above, namely the invasion of the
husband's proprietorial rights in his wife, would not have much
force in a modern developed society; in such a society a wife is not
regarded as a piece of property. Even if this was accepted it would

not be a ground for condemning consensual AID, but it could be used to condemn AID undertaken without the husband's consent.

Adultery was also disapproved of, because it might make the husband jealous and perhaps result in the wife's affection being transferred to a third party.

It has been suggested that where a woman undergoes AID, even with the consent of her husband, she might form some kind of psychological attachment to the donor, but, there is no evidence that this is either widespread or serious. It must be borne in mind that the donor's identity is not known to the woman and there is no sexual gratification. This applies both to consensual and non-consensual AID. There is in addition some evidence that marriages in which consensual AID has been undertaken are more stable than average.

It has been noted that a social stigma may attach to a woman who has committed adultery and to her husband. The same stigma may attach where a woman undergoes AID without her husband's consent. It is however unlikely that this will be so if the husband has been a willing participant in the process. A couple's involvement with AID is regarded by the medical practitioner as confidential and couples do not seem willing to publicize the fact that they have had AID. Even if AID was more commonly known there is no evidence that consensual AID would be disapproved of.

One point about adultery which was stressed in almost all the above comments is the risk that it will introduce into the family children who have no blood link with the husband. This argument reflects a concern about purity of blood, which in turn is associated with succession to estates and the former emphasis on inheritance by legitimate children. Although in the past illegitimate children have been discriminated against in law, the position has altered radically and the legal differences between legitimate and illegitimate children in the UK have largely disappeared. The social stigma which attached to illegitimacy has also diminished.

If a couple are concerned about purity of blood and hence legitimacy AID will not be acceptable to them. Conversely any couple contemplating AID would not be likely to be unduly concerned about this matter. Where AID is undertaken with the husband's consent the children born as the result are not the husband's children. The important point however is that he is not deceived into thinking that they are his. Even in the case where the woman undergoes AID without her husband's consent he is not necessarily deceived, because she may freely admit that she has had AID.

The last ground on which adultery is condemned is that it may adversely affect the stability of the family. It has been observed that the family is 'the fundamental instrumental foundation of the larger social structure, in that all other institutions depend upon its contribution.'[25] The contributions made by the family are said to include economic, socializing, sexual and reproductive functions. In addition it provides education for its members and gives them a particular status within society.[26] Given the importance of the family, anything which might affect the ways in which it functions must be carefully examined. In considering AID, it is clear that the sexual and reproductive functions of the family are of paramount significance.

The fact that a woman undergoes AID does not remove the sexual function from the family, in that the parties can continue to have intercourse, but it does involve, at least for the male, the removal of the reproductive function. It is difficult to know whether that would have, or has had, any effect on families, because if the husband is incapable of producing children he will be forced to come to terms with that, even if his wife does not undergo AID. Some couples may regret having had AID but for others it may be a means of transforming an unhappy childless marriage into a happy, and perhaps more stable, unit. Some statistics demonstrate that the divorce rate among childless couples is higher than average,[27] whereas there is some evidence that the rate of marital breakdown among AID couples is lower than average.[28] This suggests that the potential parents have been skilfully selected and that any misgivings or psychological attachments or jealousies have been overcome.

These observations presuppose that AID is practised primarily in order to overcome infertility. However it may also be undertaken to prevent the transmission of an inheritable defect to a child. This would not affect the stability of the family, any more than would its use to overcome infertility.

Nevertheless AID might be seen as a threat to the family, if it was widely available to unmarried women or was used to eliminate 'undesirable' characteristics and produce other traits which society or geneticists regarded as 'desirable' – what has been called eutelegenesis. This use of AID is the central theme of Aldous Huxley's *Brave New World* and was advocated by the Nobel Prize-winner Dr Hermann Muller.[29] Dr Muller's ideas have not yet been implemented, but in the United States there are semen banks which give fairly extensive details of the donors and some of these permit postal applications. Furthermore – and this is nearer to Muller's notion – there is a bank in Los Angeles where the donors are all said to be Nobel Prize-winners or other outstanding individuals.[30] The operators of the bank have denied that it is their intention to produce superior individuals,[31] but the first child to be born (called

Doron) was estimated to have an IQ of 200 at the age of four months.[32]

Any attempt to ascertain the purposes underlying the divorce provisions on adultery, and to apply these to AID, meets with certain obstacles. The first is that although a statute may say that if a spouse commits adultery the other may petition for divorce, there may be little or nothing to indicate why that society disapproves of adultery, and the reasons vary. The second is that because in the majority of instances AID is carried out only after full consultation with the husband and with his consent, some of the reasons for the opposition to adultery are irrelevant. Thus while one may oppose adultery because it may deceive the husband into thinking that children born to his wife are his children, this argument cannot be used where AID is undertaken with his consent. However it may be argued that if adultery can affect the stability of a family unit, AID may have the same effect; but the effects of AID have not been examined in detail and there is little evidence one way or the other. One has to rely almost entirely on information from any practitioners who attempt to follow up the patient, her husband and the child. That evidence does not support the view that AID results in unstable marriages.

The last problem is that the use of definitions to identify the purposes underlying divorce provisions cannot be applied without qualifications to AID, because the law was developed without having AID in mind. While Orde, J. in the case of *Orford v. Orford* already mentioned tried to analyse adultery and AID, what he was really doing was making a policy decision that AID was wrong and should be condemned in the same way as adultery. Because of the similarity which adultery has to non-consensual AID, he attempted to extend the definition of the one to encompass the other.

Possible approaches by the courts to non-consensual AID

Against that background we can look at the cases in which AID has been considered by the courts, and their approaches to the issue, whether any changes have been suggested and finally whether reform is best achieved by legislation or the courts.

Where a court has to consider non-consensual AID in a divorce action where there are specified grounds, it may say that it does not amount to adultery or any of the other grounds, and that any gap can be filled only by legislation. Alternatively the court may say that, while such conduct is not exactly covered by the grounds for divorce, the intention of the legislature was to provide a remedy in the circumstances.

The reported cases

The earliest reported case is the Canadian *Orford v. Orford*[33] referred to above. A newly-married couple spent their honeymoon in England but failed to consummate their marriage because the wife experienced pain while attempting to have intercourse. Her husband returned to Canada alone, leaving his wife to undergo treatment and she returned to Canada six years later. When the husband refused to have her back she initiated proceedings for alimony. His defence was that she had committed adultery and given birth to a child. The wife insisted that she had consulted a doctor who prescribed AID as a remedy for her sexual problems and that she had conceived the child as a result. The court concluded that the wife had committed adultery and held that the husband was justified in resisting his wife's claim for maintenance. The finding of adultery was sufficient to dispose of the matter; but Orde mentioned the AID and held that a woman who gives birth to a child as the result of AID is guilty of adultery:

> The term 'adultery', has never had an exact meaning, nor has its meaning been the same in all countries or under all systems of law, but all the definitions, whatever be the system of law, or whatever the country . . . use the term 'sexual intercourse', or some synonymous expression to describe one of the necessary ingredients of adultery.

The wife argued that without sexual intercourse there could not be adultery, but that was rejected because, in the judge's opinion, it showed the fallacy of relying on a definition without having regard to the branch of law of which it formed a part. He then continued:

> It is admitted that there is no direct authority upon the exact point . . . The sin or offence of adultery, as affecting the marriage, may be traced from the Mosaic Law down through the canon or ecclesiastical law to the present date . . . In its essence, adultery was an invasion of the marital rights of the husband and wife . . . Can anyone read the Mosaic Law . . . without being convinced that had such a thing as artificial insemination entered the mind of the law-giver, it would have been regarded with the utmost horror as an invasion of the most sacred rights of husband and wife, and have been the subject of the severest penalties? . . . the essence of the offence of adultery consists . . . in the voluntary surrender to another person of the reproductive powers or faculties of the guilty person.

These observations have been criticized earlier and there is no need to repeat what has been said. The decision is probably best classified as one of policy. Since the decision in *Orford v. Orford* there have been four other cases on this point, three American and one Scottish. The American decisions are *Hoch v. Hoch*,[34] *Doornbos v.*

Doornbos[35] and *People v. Sorensen;*[36] and the Scottish case is *MacLennan v. MacLennan.*[37]

In *Hoch v. Hoch*, a Chicago case, the husband returned home after two years of military service. His wife was pregnant and he raised an action for divorce on the grounds of adultery. The wife's defence was that she had undergone AID, but the court held that she had committed adultery. The judge went on to say that if the wife had proved that she had had AID, that would not have amounted to adultery.

In the later case of *Doornbos v. Doornbos*, also in Chicago, the opposite conclusion was reached. A wife had been granted a divorce on the ground of the husband's habitual drunkenness. There was a child which the wife said had been conceived as the result of AID to which the husband had given his consent, and that was not contradicted by the husband. The wife asked the court to decide whether AID amounted to adultery. The trial judge made the following pronouncement:

> 1. Heterologous artificial insemination (when the specimen of semen used is obtained from a third party or donor) with or without the consent of the husband, is contrary to public policy and good morals, and constitutes adultery on the part of the mother. A child so conceived is not a child born in wedlock and therefore illegitimate. As such it is the child of the mother and the father [sic] has no right or interest in the said child.
> 2. Homologous artificial insemination (when the specimen of semen used is obtained from the husband of the woman) is not contrary to public policy and good morals, and does not present any difficulty from the legal point of view.

An appeal was dismissed on purely procedural grounds, and the appeal court did not comment on these observations.

The last American case, *People v. Sorensen*, was a criminal case in California, in which the issue was whether a husband was obliged to support a child conceived by AID to which he had consented. The facts were that the husband was sterile and after fifteen years of unsuccessful attempts to produce a child, he agreed that his wife should undergo AID. For over four years after the birth of the child a normal family relationship existed, but then the parties separated. Mrs Sorensen told her husband she would consent to a divorce and would not ask for maintenance for the child. A divorce was granted, but two years later Mrs Sorensen became ill and was forced to apply for public assistance. The local district attorney demanded that Mr Sorensen pay for the child's support, and when he failed to do so he was prosecuted under the Californian Penal Code and was convicted. The leading judgment was given by Justice McComb who dealt with the issue of adultery, saying:

In the absence of legislation prohibiting artificial insemination, the offspring of defendant's valid marriage to the child's mother was lawfully begotten and was not the product of an illicit or adulterous relationship. Adultery is defined as 'the voluntary sexual intercourse of a married person with a person other than the offender's husband or wife'. It has been suggested that the doctor and the wife commit adultery by the process of artificial insemination. Since the doctor may be a woman, or the husband himself may administer the insemination by a syringe, this is patently absurd; to consider it an act of adultery with the donor, who at the time of insemination may be a thousand miles away or may even be dead, is equally absurd.

The last reported case, and the only decision in the United Kingdom, is the Scottish case of *MacLennan v. MacLennan*, decided in 1958. This case raised the issue whether AID without the husband's consent amounts to adultery. The parties were married in 1952, but they had not lived together since early 1954. The wife admitted that on 10 July 1955 she had given birth to a child in New York and for that reason the husband wanted to divorce her on the grounds of adultery. The wife's defence was that the child had been conceived as the result of AID. She did not allege that the husband had consented and he maintained that he had never agreed to the process. Her argument, however, was that AID, even without her husband's consent, was not adultery in Scots law. Lord Wheatley agreed, saying:

> It is almost trite to say that a married woman who, without the consent of her husband, has the seed of a male donor injected into her person by mechanical means, in order to procreate a child who would not be the child of the marriage, has committed a grave and heinous breach of the contract of marriage. The question for my determination, however, is not the moral culpability of such an act, but is whether such an act constitutes adultery in its legal meaning . . . If it is not adultery, although a grave breach of the marriage contract, that is a matter for the Legislature if it be thought that a separate legal remedy should be provided.

He also said that to determine what was meant by adultery one had to look at leading legal writers or reported decisions. He referred to a number of authorities, especially English ones, and said:

> I have quoted these English cases at some length, since it seems possible to derive therefrom the following propositions, according at least to the law of England:
>
> 1. For adultery to be committed there must be the two parties physically present and the engaging in the sexual act at the same time.
> 2. To constitute the sexual act there must be an act of union involving some degree of penetration of the female organ by the male organ.

3. It is not a necessary concomitant of adultery that male seed should be deposited in the female's ovum.
4. The placing of the male seed in the female ovum need not necessarily result from the sexual act, and if it does not, but is placed there by some other means, there is no sexual intercourse.

I can find nothing to persuade me that the law of Scotland is not the same as the law of England so far as the legal propositions above enunciated are concerned . . . and in my opinion these propositions are equally valid in our law . . . If my views be correct, then it follows logically that artificial insemination by a donor without the consent of the husband is not adultery as the law interprets that term.

He continued:

It is perhaps not inappropriate, however, to consider the implications of the contrary view. If artificial insemination by a donor without the husband's consent is to be deemed adultery, the first question which seems to call for a decision is whether the donor whose seed has been used has himself been guilty of adultery. If the answer is in the affirmative, the further question arises, at what point of time has he done so? If it be at the point when the seed is extracted from his body, certain interesting considerations would arise. I gather that the seed so obtained can be retained for a considerable time before being used, and in some cases it may not be used at all. If the donor's seed is taken merely to lie *in retentis*, it surely cannot be adultery if that seed is never used. Thus, if his adultery is to be deemed to take place at the time of the parting with the seed, it can only be an adultery subject to defeasance in the event of the seed not being used. Such a statement need only be stated for its absurdity to be manifested. If, on the other hand, his adultery is deemed to take place when the seed is injected into the woman's ovum, this latter act may take place after his death, and in that case the woman's conduct would constitute not only adultery but necrophilism. Such a proposition seems to me to be equally absurd. The third alternative is that the whole process should be regarded as an act of adultery, but as this might in certain cases result in the act covering a period of say two years, and be committed partly during the lifetime and partly after the death of the donor, I cannot distinguish between the absurdity of such a proposition and the absurdity of the other alternatives. Senior counsel for the pursuer appreciated the illogicality and absurdity of these consequences of the proposition that the donor had committed adultery, and accepted that he had not. This then forced him to argue that the wife could commit adultery by herself. One need not consider the interesting point whether the administrator could be said to commit adultery, because the administrator might be a woman or the seed might be self-injected by the wife herself operating the syringe. The idea that a woman is committing adultery when alone in the privacy of her bedroom she injects into her ovum by means of a syringe the seed of a man she does not know and has never seen is one which I am afraid I cannot accept. Unilateral adultery is possible, as in the case of a married man who ravages a woman not his wife, but self-adultery is a conception as yet unknown to the law.

He then said that it was up to the wife to establish that the child had been conceived as a result of AID and that her failure to do so would result in an inference of adultery. Although the wife was given the opportunity to provide the necessary information, she failed to do so and so the divorce was granted.

These decisions clearly demonstrate the different approaches to AID. In *Orford v. Orford* Orde J.'s decision was really one of policy – that the definition of adultery covered non-consensual AID. In *Doornbos v. Doornbos* the decision was also one of policy – that even where the husband consented AID still amounted to adultery. In the cases of Sorensen and MacLennan, the judges reached their decisions partly by analysing various definitions, but they also made some observations on policy. In *People v. Sorensen* the judge said that because there was no legislation which prohibited AID a child which was born during the husband's marriage was legitimate. In *MacLennan v. MacLennan* Lord Wheatley was also faced with a set of circumstances which were not covered by legislation, but he left it to legislation to fill the gap if necessary.

There have of course been comments by academic writers on this subject, but many of these have done no more than examine the definitions and reported decisions. Most of them have concluded that AID does not amount to adultery, and one writer has recently put the matter forcibly: 'Identification of AID with adultery can no longer seriously be maintained'.[38] A few commentators have suggested that AID without the consent of the husband could amount to cruelty.[39] Others have proposed changes in the law which would regulate both consensual and non-consensual AID, but they have either expressly or by implication left the initiative with the legislature rather than entrust it to the courts.[40]

Conclusion

There can be little doubt that the law on this aspect of AID requires clarification in many jurisdictions. The important question is how a court ought to react when the issue of AID comes before it in divorce proceedings. Given the traditional approach to the interpretation of the terms 'adultery' and 'sexual intercourse', it is unlikely that courts will conclude that AID without the husband's consent amounts in law to adultery. If the courts are unable to reach that conclusion, they may still say that such conduct amounts to cruelty or its equivalent. For example, in the UK the courts could grant a divorce on the basis that a woman who receives AID without her husband's consent has behaved in such a way that her husband cannot reasonably be expected to continue to live with her. Of course if divorce is available on more general grounds, such as irretrievable breakdown of marriage, it would probably be easier to bring non-consensual AID within the divorce framework than it would be where the grounds for divorce are more detailed.

If none of these courses is open the courts may approach the problem in one of two ways. They may take the course chosen by Orde J. and decide that it was the intention of the divorce provisions to include non-consensual AID, which is a policy approach, or follow Lord Wheatley, saying that the problem was not susceptible of a solution within the existing framework, and perhaps combine that with a suggestion that there should be legislation to clarify the position.

The remaining question is which of these two courses is preferable. We would support the latter, for a number of reasons. The first is that while a decision by a judge that non-consensual AID may be within the intended ambit of the divorce law, non-consensual AID is rarely practised and therefore the position of couples practising consensual AID would remain uncertain.

A second reason is that, while a decision that non-consensual AID is adultery will determine the status of the child born as a result, it would not decide the status of a child born as a result of AID where the husband has consented.

The final, and perhaps most compelling, reason is that any statement of policy should cover all aspects of the subject and not just the legal ones. These include the attitude of the medical profession and the psychological implications, for example the ways in which AID affects the couple, the child, the donor and the physician. There are also ethical, religious and sociological issues. Few, if any, judges are competent to pronounce on all of these issues, and even if they were it seems unlikely that they would be provided with the necessary evidence to make the decision. Even if a judge tackled the question of policy, his judgment might not be binding upon judges outside his jurisdiction, and within his jurisdiction other judges might feel free to disregard any utterances on matters which were not central to the case.

The usual and most satisfactory way of obtaining information with a view to formulating policy is to appoint a commission of inquiry. This was done in relation to artificial insemination in 1958 when the government appointed the Feversham Committee, and again in 1982 when the Warnock Committee was set up to consider artificial insemination and other techniques which had developed since the 1960s.

Egg donation and embryo donation

What has been said about AID and adultery applies equally to egg donation. If it were accepted that AID, whether consensual or not, is adultery, egg donation would also be adultery, this time however by the husband. It follows therefore that embryo donation would be adultery by both husband and wife.

Although the previous pages have attempted to refute the argument that AID is adultery, both egg donation and embryo donation performed without the consent of the husband would be grounds for divorce in the UK. It is highly improbable however that this issue would even arise.

7 Maintenance, custody and succession rights of AID children

As has been said, the status of the child born as the result of AID may determine, or have some bearing upon, questions of maintenance, custody and succession. Other terms such as 'support' and 'ailment' may be used rather than 'maintenance'.

In most jurisdictions a father is under a legal obligation to support his biological child. This obligation arises at birth and continues until the child reaches an age at which the law regards it as being able to look after itself. One reason for imposing this duty is that support and protection are needed to bring children to an age of maturity and it prevents them being a burden on the community. The obligation has always been imposed on the biological father because he was responsible for bringing the child into existence, and as a result he was given custody of the child. Rights of succession would follow naturally from those other rights and obligations, but for succession purposes sons, and particularly the eldest son, would in the past have had a preference, as they were regarded as more suitable substitutes for the father in a war and in exercising control over the other members of the family.

Maintenance and Custody

At one time in Scotland, and in Anglo-American jurisdictions, maintenance and custody were determined by the child's status. On that basis a legitimate child would be entitled to be maintained by its father and the father would be entitled to custody of the child. If therefore an AID child were regarded as the husband's legitimate child, then he and not the donor would be obliged to provide for it and would be entitled to custody. On the other hand, if the AID child were regarded as illegitimate, while it might have rights against its mother and certain obligations might be imposed on her,

her husband would not have any rights nor would he be under any obligation even to maintain the child. Any rights and obligations would be the donor's as the biological father, even if he could not be identified.

Although that was the position at common law, a number of jurisdictions have departed from the traditional approach, either by judicial decision or legislation.

United States

As with many other aspects of AID, the main legal activity has been in the USA.

The first case, *Strnad v. Strnad*, was heard in New York in 1948.[1] A husband who was legally separated from his wife claimed visitation rights in respect of a child born as the result of AID, to which he was assumed to have given his consent. The wife resisted her husband's claim, asserting that the child was not his child. The court took the view that the husband was entitled to visitation rights because that was in the best interests of the child. It was held that the child had been potentially adopted or semi-adopted, and that it was not in a different position from a child which had been legitimized by the subsequent marriage of its parents.

Later in Illinois in the case of *Doornbos v. Doornbos*[2] a wife raised an action for divorce on the ground of her husband's habitual drunkenness. During the hearing she sought a ruling on the status of a child which had been born as the result of AID to which her husband had given his consent and in respect of which the husband was asking for visitation rights. In this case the court held that the child was illegitimate. It denied the husband's request for visitation rights and relieved him of any obligations of support. However, at the request of the trial judge, the State Attorney filed a petition on behalf of the State of Illinois to reverse that part of the decision which relieved the husband of any obligation to support the child.

The State's argument was that a finding of illegitimacy deprived the child of rights of support and inheritance, and further that if the mother failed to support the child the State would be forced to do so, since it would be *in loco parentis*. Because the trial judge refused to alter his decision the State took the issue to the Appellate Court, but the appeal was dismissed on purely procedural grounds. The approach of the court of first instance was more traditional than that adopted in *Strnad v. Strnad*. Having held that the child was illegitimate, that in turn determined the issue of visitation.

In another New York case, *People ex rel Abajian v. Dennett*[3], the husband sought custody of the children. The wife argued that as they had been conceived as the result of AID they were not the husband's children, and accordingly he was not entitled to either custody or visitation rights. However the court decided that by her subsequent conduct the wife had treated her husband as the children's parent and it refused to allow her to bring evidence about the circumstances in which they were conceived. Although this case involved AID children and questions of custody and visitation, it is not very helpful, since the decision was reached without any comment on the main issues, in particular on whether the fact that a child had been born as the result of AID affected visitation rights.

A much more instructive decision is that in *Gursky v. Gursky*,[4] again a New York case, in which a husband agreed to his wife undergoing AID and agreed to pay all the expenses of her treatment. In a subsequent divorce action the wife asked for support for the child, but the husband denied that he was under any obligation in respect of it. The court held that AID amounted to adultery, but because the husband had consented to the AID he was liable to support the child. The court based its decision on two grounds – implied consent and equitable estoppel. By giving his consent to the AID, the husband was impliedly agreeing to provide for any child which might be born as the result. Furthermore the consent form narrated that the couple wished the physician to embark on AID for the express purpose of providing a child for the 'natural happiness' of the couple. The court therefore held that the wife had been induced by the husband to alter her position to her detriment. Accordingly, to relieve the husband of any duty to provide support would put the burden on the wife and the court regarded that as inequitable because the wife had undergone AID in reliance on the husband's wishes – equitable estoppel.

In *Anon. v. Anon.*,[5] which was decided the year after *Gursky v. Gursky* and in the same jurisdiction, a wife sought support from her husband for an AID child. The husband had given written consent and again the court took the view that he had consented to provide support for the child.

Our final case, the Californian *People v. Sorensen*,[6] was a criminal prosecution of a husband who had failed to provide support for an AID child where he had consented to its conception. The local district attorney required Sorensen to pay for the child's support and, when he refused, he was prosecuted under s.270 of the Californian Penal Code and was convicted. The relevant provision was:

A father of either a legitimate or illegitimate minor child . . . who wilfully omits without lawful excuse to furnish necessary clothing, food, shelter or medical attendance or other remedial care for his child is guilty of a misdemeanour . . .

Sorensen successfully appealed to the Court of Appeal, but the conviction was restored by the California Supreme Court. It is however instructive to look briefly at the approach taken by the appeal court.

Justice Devine who delivered the judgment emphasized that it was for the prosecution to prove that Sorensen was 'the father' of the child, and he held that it had failed. The lower court had proceeded on the basis of estoppel which meant that because Sorensen had consented to the artificial insemination and had accepted the child for four years as a part of the family, he could not at a later stage deny that he was the father. Estoppel or bar is a civil law concept and Justice Devine observed that there were no criminal cases where estoppel had been used to make certain conduct a crime.

The Supreme Court unanimously restored the conviction. Justice McComb who delivered the judgment of the court proceeded on the basis of the presumption of paternity which arose where a married woman gave birth to a child. He held that that presumption could not be overcome unless there was scientific evidence that the husband was sterile, and he held that for the purposes of s.270, Sorensen was 'the lawful father'. The section was not concerned with the biological father and because a child conceived as a result of AID did not have a 'natural' father, the husband who gave his consent was the lawful father. In the court's view the donor of semen made no greater contribution than a blood donor. One further point made by the court was that Mrs Sorensen could not surrender the child's right to support.

Two points are worth making about the decisions in these cases. The first is that the courts were always faced with a situation in which the husband had given his consent to AID, or was presumed to have given it, and where, at least for some time, the child was brought up as a member of the family. In such cases it is easier to hold that the husband has impliedly agreed to provide for the child, or that he is barred from refusing to support it, or that he is presumed to be the father. As yet no court has imposed an obligation of support on a husband who has not given consent to AID. In such a case the doctrine of implied consent would clearly be inapplicable. It might be possible to found on equitable estoppel or bar if, subsequent to the birth, the husband had treated the child as his own and had induced his wife to believe that he would continue to support it. That might have influenced the court in *Strnad v. Strnad*, where it was decided that it was in the best interests of the child to receive support from the husband. It may be however that there is no subsequent conduct on the part of the husband which would permit such a decision. The second point is that there did not seem to be any contradiction in saying that the child was illegitimate, but that the husband was nevertheless under an obligation to support it or was entitled to visitation rights.

In the absence of statutory provisions specifically dealing with the AID child, the legal position in the USA is somewhat uncertain, even where the husband gives his consent. In most of the cases he has been held liable for support and, while this may seem a sensible solution where the husband has consented to the AID, there can be no certainty that, in future, courts will be persuaded to adopt this approach, rather than the view taken in *Doornbos v. Doornbos* that the husband had no rights in the child and vice versa.

United Kingdom

Until recently the UK did not have legislation in respect of children conceived by AID. At common law the husband would not be under any obligation to maintain such a child, whether or not he had given his consent to the insemination.

There are however statutory provisions which alleviate this harshness where the child has been accepted as a member of the husband's family. The Matrimonial Proceedings (Children) Act 1958,[7] which applies to Scotland, and the Matrimonial Causes Act 1973,[8] which applies to England and Wales, provide that in actions for divorce, nullity and separation the courts may make an order for the maintenance of a child of the family. Under the Domestic Proceedings and Magistrates Courts Act 1978, which again applies only to England and Wales, either party to a marriage may apply to the magistrates court for reasonable maintenance for such a child.[9] In Scotland under the Family Law (Scotland) Act 1985, there is a general obligation to provide aliment (maintenance) for such children.[10]

Beneficial as such legislation is, what is really required in respect of the AID child is a statute which recognizes that the consenting husband is in law the father of the child for all purposes.

Succession

There do not seem to be any reported decisions in the USA or UK on the succession rights of an AID child. In both the *Strnad* and the *Gursky* cases the courts expressly declined to discuss the matter, but any decision, such as *Doornbos v. Doornbos*, which declares the AID child to be illegitimate, may by implication determine the question of inheritance, namely that the child is not entitled to succeed to the husband's estate unless specifically provided for in a will. However, while the court in *Doornbos v. Doornbos* stated that the husband had no rights or interest in the child, in *Gursky v. Gursky* the court did no more than hold that the child was illegitimate.

If there are no specific statutory provisions on the subject, and there are none in the UK, the AID child's rights of succession lie against the estate of the donor as the biological father, rather than the husband. Even statutory provisions which allow illegitimate children to succeed to the estate of their natural parents would not assist in the case of an AID child, as its natural parents would be the mother and the donor, not the husband.

Legislation

Most of the legislation on this issue has been passed in the USA. The first enactment was in Georgia in 1964 and later legislation has largely followed that pattern. The relevant part of the Georgia code is as follows:

> All children born within wedlock or within the usual period of gestation thereafter, who have been conceived by means of artificial insemination, are irrevocably presumed legitimate if both the husband and the wife consent in writing to the use and administration of artificial insemination.[11]

In Chapter 8 mention is made of certain problems which this type of provision creates, for example the effect of absence of consent, and the fact that most of the enactments are not retrospective. There is no need to anticipate what is said there. What is clear is that, if the conditions laid down in the statute are complied with, the child will be the legitimate child of the husband, and so it will have exactly the same rights in the husband's estate as any other legitimate child, and any rights which it might have against the donor and vice versa would cease to exist. Because there is no such legislation in the UK it is by no means certain that, in every situation, the AID child will succeed to the husband's estate.

In two situations however there is legislation. In England and Wales (but not Scotland) under the Inheritance of Family and Dependants Act 1975, a child which has been brought up as a member of the family by a person will be able to claim against the estate on his death if no other provision has been made, for example in a will.[12] The other situation is covered by section 27 of the Family Law Reform Act 1987 referred to earlier in this chapter. However, because it, like the 1975 Act, applies only in England and Wales, an AID child would not succeed to its social father should he die intestate, because the child would not be his illegitimate child.

Where the husband leaves a will providing for 'my children' or 'my issue' these words now include illegitimate children in both England and Wales and Scotland.[13] If the AID child was regarded as legitimate it would succeed to the husband's estate, but if it was illegitimate it would not be covered by either the term 'children' or 'issue' since it would be the donor's illegitimate child and the child therefore could be at a serious disadvantage.

The statutory provision does not sever any legal links which the AID child has with the donor. While it is unlikely that the donor's identity would be known to the child or that he could find out who the donor was, if there was no legislation to the contrary the child could have a right to succeed to the donor's estate as one of his illegitimate children.

If the donor left a will in which he referred to 'my children' or 'my issue' these phrases might be interpreted as including illegitimate children. Even where the donor died intestate some jurisdictions, including those in the UK, recognize a right of illegitimate children to share in their parents' estates.

It is perhaps fortunate that AID children cannot identify the donors with a view to making claims on their estates as this would give rise to enormous problems. For example, the donor's estate could not safely be wound up until all possible claimants had been identified. Indeed it is difficult to see how, in some cases, a donor's estate could ever be wound up if his semen was in a sperm bank and was still being used after his death. As with status, an almost incontrovertible case is made out for severing all legal links between the donor and the child and making the husband the father for all purposes.

Children conceived by egg donation   The law outlined above applies equally where a child is conceived from a donor egg. In that situation however the child's legal ties would be with the husband (the father) and the ovum donor. However if the husband's wife (assuming a married couple are the recipients) had brought the child up as hers she would be liable to maintain it, and the 1975 Act would assist such a child if the wife did not make any satisfactory provision for it in her will.

Children conceived by embryo donation   In this situation the child's legal ties are with the donors and not with either the husband or the wife (assuming again that a married couple are the recipients). Once again, however, both could be liable for maintenance and the child could have a right under the 1975 Act.

8 Status of the AID child

One of the issues which may concern a married couple contemplating AID is whether the child will be regarded in law as the husband's child. The legal position of the child will determine how its birth ought to be registered but, more importantly, it will determine whether it has a right to succeed to the husband's estate on his death. These points are clearly important for the couple but they have implications for other people, for example the couple's relatives, and for society as a whole. They arise also in egg donation and embryo donation and what is said here applies also there.

In many systems of law, including those of the UK, the USA, France, West Germany, and Canada, there are a number of different statuses for children. The main ones are legitimate children, illegitimate children and adopted children. The rights enjoyed by children will to a great extent depend on the legal relationship with their parents. In these legal systems, for example, illegitimate children enjoy fewer rights than legitimate children, although the differences are not as marked as they once were.

Many statutory changes have been made to the common law position, but even with these changes there are still differences between the legal positions, depending upon the jurisdiction. The status of adopted children was not known to the common law and so the rights which these children have are laid down by statute.[1]

Legitimate children enjoy the fullest rights and it is against these that the rights of other children are measured. At common law a child was legitimate if it was born of a legally valid marriage. The approach of the Anglo–American legal systems was that 'the only person who could claim to be legitimate was one born in lawful wedlock arising from a marriage of a Christian nature'.[2] Thus there was an emphasis on monogamous marriage, concern for its stability and an aversion to any relationship which might result in the birth of an illegitimate child.[3]

At common law the illegitimate child (sometimes called *filius nullius* or *filius populi*) possessed few rights and was subject to many restrictions principally in connection with maintenance and succession.[4] In the present century however there have been significant changes. As one distinguished House of Lords judge, Lord Reid, said,

> In former times it was plainly in the child's interest to have a finding of legitimacy even where the presumption of legitimacy had been used to overcome evidence which without it would have pointed the other way. An illegitmate child was not only deprived of the financial advantage of legitimacy but in most circles of society, other than those considered disreputable, it carried throughout its life a stigma which made it a second class citizen. But now modern legislation has removed almost all the financial disadvantages of illegitmacy and it has become difficult to foretell how grave a handicap the stigma of illegitimacy will prove to be in later life. There are two aspects to this; how far will its neighbours look down on the child by reason of its illegitimacy and how far will the child itself feel a sense of inferiority? Doubtless there are still many circles where an illegitmate person is not well received. But there are many others, particularly in large towns, where nobody knows and nobody cares whether a newcomer is legitimate or illegitimate, and one hopes that prejudice against a person unfortunate enough to be illegitmate is decreasing.[5]

Although he was referring in the main to the social consequences of illegitimacy, in a number of jurisdictions the legal position of illegitimate children has also been improved. Statutory provisions have introduced recognition or acknowledgement by the natural father, and adoption, and certain children have been declared legitimate even though their parents were not married or not validly married.[6] In general however considerable stress is still put on whether a child is legitimate or not. In the absence of statutory provisions such as those mentioned above, that will depend on whether its parents were married at the time of its conception.[7]

One could say that an AID child is not the husband's child and so cannot be legitimate. However, where a couple are validly married and a child is born to the wife there is a legal presumption that the woman's husband is the father of the child,[8] and an AID child would have the benefit of that presumption.

Some legal writers have regrettably made the issue more complex by comparing AID with adultery in an attempt to define the status of the AID child.[9] This can be seen clearly from one analysis:

> Whether a child born as a result of artificial insemination is legitimate depends upon whether his mother's impregnation constituted adultery. If so, the child conceived is illegitimate; if not, the offspring's legitimacy cannot be questioned.[10]

If this is accurate it would follow that, although there was clear evidence that the child had been conceived as the result of AID, it would not be illegitimate unless AID also amounts in law to adultery. Putting it another way, the child would be legitimate even though there was clear evidence that the husband was not the father.

If it can be shown that a child has been conceived in adultery it will be illegitimate. Likewise if it can be shown that it was conceived by AID it will be illegitmate. The reason in both cases is that the semen did not come from the husband, but it is not necessary to equate AID with adultery to reach that conclusion. If a married woman gives birth to an AID child then it is presumed in law to be the husband's child (and he will usually register it as such). Although the presumption will be difficult to rebut, it can be overcome, for example by proof of the husband's sterility or non-access to his wife during the period when the child was conceived. That will be almost impossible, because the couple's involvement with AID will usually be known only to the husband, the wife and the medical practitioner and, in most cases, none of them will wish to prove that the husband may not be the father. One says 'may' because there will remain in some cases the possibility, albeit remote, that the husband is the father.

However if the couple separate or obtain a divorce the wife may wish to deprive her husband of rights in the child or the husband may not want to be obliged to maintain it. In order to succeed they would have to show that the child was conceived as the result of AID; but they may not succeed for a number of reasons. In some jurisdictions 'parents' will not be permitted to give evidence, which might bastardize the child.[11] As was said in one American case, 'to stigmatize them as children of an unknown father by means of artificial insemination of the mother is no more . . . than an attempt to make these innocents out as children of bastardy. And where a parent attempts such means, the law will seal the lips of such a parent.'[12]

Other factors may also make proof difficult. For example, the husband may have had intercourse with his wife while she was undergoing AID,[13] or the medical practitioner may have mixed the husband's semen with that of the donor[14] or matched the blood group of the donor with that of the husband.[15] In any event, the wife may find it difficult to obtain evidence from her husband's medical practitioner about his condition, because he will regard the relationship between him and his patient as confidential and will probably refuse to disclose the information unless he is required by a court to do so.[16] If these obstacles are overcome the child will be declared illegitimate, but if the husband has treated the child as his, in some jurisdictions he will be under an obligation to maintain it.

The approaches to the issue of the status of the AID child noted so far recognize that if a child is conceived during marriage it will be presumed legitimate. The alternative is to declare the child illegitimate if the presumption is overcome.

There are however two other approaches. One is to hold that, although a child conceived as the result of AID is illegitimate, the special circumstances of its conception and upbringing require that it should be treated as if it were the legitimate offspring of the husband. The second is simply to declare that an AID child is legitimate. At this point it is instructive to look again at some of the cases in the USA which have been considered earlier.

There are five decisions which consider the status of the AID child. The first, *Strnad v. Strnad*,[17] was decided in 1948. A wife who had obtained a divorce from her husband was granted custody of a child which had been conceived as the result of AID to which her husband had consented. The husband was granted visitation rights (access), but the wife later attempted to have these withdrawn on the basis that the child was illegitimate. The court held that the child was 'potentially adopted' or 'semi-adopted', and was not illegitimate. The judge said: '[L]ogically and realistically, the situation is no different than that pertaining in the case of a child born out of wedlock who by law is made legitimate upon the marriage of the interested parties.'[18] Although these terms do not have a special meaning in law, the judge clearly thought that it was inequitable to regard an AID child as illegitimate and so his decision was based on what he thought ought to be the State's policy.

A completely different result was reached in *Doornbos v. Doornbos*,[19] where a woman was granted a divorce but wanted custody of a child. According to her evidence, which was not contradicted, it had been conceived as the result of AID to which her husband had consented. However she contended that the child was illegitimate and that she alone was entitled to custody. The trial judge held that AID was contrary to public policy and said: 'A child so conceived is not a child born in wedlock, and therefore is illegitimate. As such, it is the child of the mother, and the father [*sic*] has no right or interest in said child.'[20] He also gave his views on policy, but his decision was really based on the traditional approach which was that if the husband was not the father the child was illegitimate. There was an appeal but the appeal court did not express any different view on the subject. Perhaps they felt that it was for the legislature and not the judges to change the law.

The matter came before another New York court in 1963 in the case of *Gursky v. Gursky*.[21] This was an action for annulment of a marriage, but the wife asked for maintenance for a child which had been conceived as the result of AID to which the husband had consented, and it had been registered as a child of the couple. The court's basic finding was that the child was illegitimate.[22] However the judge went on to say that because the husband had given the consent he had impliedly promised to maintain the child. Alternatively, because the husband had persuaded his wife to undergo AID, he could not later refuse to support the child. *Gursky* is a more constructive decision than either *Strnad* or *Doornbos* in the sense that the decision reflects what was in the best interests of the child, but it was reached within the existing legal framework.

In 1973 yet another New York court was faced with the issue.[23] A woman had given birth to a child as the result of consensual AID. In divorce proceedings the child was declared legitimate. When the woman later remarried, her second husband wished to adopt the child. He argued that because it had been conceived as the result of AID the first husband was not a 'parent' and so it was not necessary to have his consent to the proposed adoption. That was rejected and the court held that the child was legitimate. The judge was influenced by New York's policy in favour of legitimacy. Recent legislation had made children born of bigamous, incestuous and adulterous relationships legitimate[24] and he could see no reason why an AID child should be stigmatized as illegitimate.[25] In this case the judge was also making a policy decision based on legislation in other areas. It is significant that the legislation did not deal with AID children, but the court nevertheless felt that it could make its own decision on policy. The court referred to the decision in *People v. Sorensen*,[26] where the court described the State's policy as being in favour of making children legitimate.

Although most of the litigation has been in the USA, at least two other courts have considered the question, one in New Zealand[27] and the other in South Africa.[28] Both courts held that the AID child was illegitimate, but in the latter case the decision was reached 'with regret'.

It is not possible to say how a particular court would approach the issues of status and maintenance where there is no legislation on the topic. In the USA the decisions have varied and have not been consistent even in the same jurisdiction. Some courts have made policy decisions, perhaps in the teeth of the strict legal position. Others have looked at the best interests of the child. The majority of courts have adopted the traditional approach and held that the AID child is illegitimate, and the fact that the husband gave his consent is irrelevant.

Scottish and English courts would probably also take this approach, but they might equally say that the husband, by giving his consent, was undertaking to provide support for the child. In both countries there is legislation about children who have been treated as members of a family, and in most cases, an AID child would come within this category.[29] The husband, therefore, could be required to maintain the child or be given access to it, perhaps even custody in preference to the mother.[30]

As noted in Chapter 7, there is legislation in England and Wales. On the husband's death a child which has been brought up as a member of his family can claim on his estate,[31] if no other reasonable provision has been made for it. There is also s.27 of the Family Law Reform Act 1987 which deals specifically with AID children, but only those born in England and Wales and not in Scotland.

Because the legal position of the AID child is uncertain there have been a number of proposals for reform,[32] but before considering these, there are two arguments which are put forward for not making any change.

Arguments against change

The first is that a change is unnecessary. Those who hold this view say that because the donor is unknown and the chances of his identity being revealed are exceedingly small it is highly unlikely that the child would be able to make any claim against him, for example for maintenance. For the same reason the donor would not be able to make any claim on the child. This approach is not convincing. It considers only the legal relationship between the donor and the child and makes no attempt to regulate the relationship between the husband and the child, which is the more important relationship and which has come before the courts. Furthermore the uncertainty in law about the husband/child relationship may tempt couples to falsify birth registers by entering the husband as the father, which would be a criminal offence.

Others who favour 'no change' take a different line. There is probably only a small minority which is of the view that the discrimination against illegitimate children, and hence AID children, is justified and should continue. This is a difficult argument to sustain, given the steps which have already been taken to alleviate the position of illegitimate children. In addition the logical consequence of the argument is that we should revert to the common law position where the illegitimate child was almost wholly disregarded. That seems unduly harsh on the children. Others, while reluctantly accepting such reform as there has been, might be opposed to any further change.

Three propositions are usually advanced for the discrimination. The first is that the legal distinction between legitimate and illegitimate children reflects social attitudes. While accepting that this *was* the case, it is no longer so. In many communities no one knows, and one suspects that few would care, whether a person is legitimate or not. Furthermore there is evidence that, in the UK at least, many illegitimate children are recognized by both parents, as can be seen from the increasing number of cases where illegitimate births are registered by both parents,[33] and a substantial number of unmarried mothers describe themselves as 'married'.[34] One extensive survey concluded that 40 per cent of illegitimate children were born into stable unions.[35]

The second argument is that the distinction between legitimate and illegitimate children supports the institution of marriage. While the institution is undoubtedly of great importance, it is clear from the increase in the number of divorces that many marriages are not stable. Those which are especially at risk are those entered into apparently to ensure that an expected child is not born illegitimate.[36] Stability of marriage is hardly reinforced by young couples entering into marriages which have little prospect of success.

The final argument is that the child's status should be determined by the legal relationship between its parents. Thus where the parents are validly married their child will be legitimate, whereas if the parents are not married then the child will be illegitimate. Not everyone would accept that it is self-evident that a child's status should be determined by the legal relationship between its parents. For example, the children of some void or voidable marriages have nevertheless been declared legitimate.[37] In the UK the child of a void marriage is legitimate if the parents mistakenly believed that the marriage was valid.[38] A child of a voidable marriage will be legitimate if it would have been legitimate on divorce.[39] The law in some of the states in the USA is similar.[40] The reason for such enactments is to avoid injustice to the children who would otherwise be visited with the 'sins' of their parents. These arguments lack cogency, but even if there is some support for them, there are features which distinguish AID from extra-marital intercourse and which justify separate provision for AID children.

There may be an ethical distinction between adultery and AID in that the latter is a clinical procedure and does not involve the mother in any personal relationship with the donor, who is anonymous and probably unaware of the insemination. Secondly where AID is undertaken the woman's husband almost invariably gives his consent, whereas this will not usually be the case with adultery. Thirdly whereas the husband may come to terms with AID and regard the child as his own, this would be less likely if the child is born as the result of adultery. Finally the fact that the husband consents to the AID probably indicates that the marriage is stable, whereas adultery usually demonstrates a lack of stability. Whether these differences have been accepted in suggestions for reform of the law, it is not easy to say.

Proposals for reform

A possible approach would be to extend the definition of 'legitimate' to the AID child, at least where the woman is married and her husband has consented to the insemination. That view was favoured by the minority of the Feversham Committee[41] and it was also adopted in a Private Member's Bill presented to parliament in 1977.[42] The minority in the Feversham Committee also thought that for the purposes of registration of births the husband should be deemed to be the father of the child. The majority of the committee however cogently argued that the law has assigned a specific meaning to the word 'legitimate' and its artificial extension to include other children would make a nonsense of the notions of status. '[T]he simple question of principle is whether a child may become the legitimate issue of those who are not his natural parents. That seems to be a contradiction in terms and the invasion of standards accepted from time immemorial.'[43] The point is well illustrated in relation to adopted children, who in many countries enjoy the same rights as legitimate children, but are not called 'legitimate'.

If this is not acceptable, the child could be given a special status, like the adopted child, which is equivalent to legitimacy; but it is difficult to think of a description of the child which would not disclose the fact that it was in some way 'different'. A more fundamental objection is that a special status could be conferred only by a legally recognized procedure, such as a petition to a court. This procedure would involve disclosing the fact that the couple had had AID, because the court would have to be satisfied that the child was entitled to the special status. For that reason alone, one suspects that many couples would avoid it. In addition if there is a possibility that the husband is the father, a new status might be given to a child where it was inappropriate. Any court procedure will take time and this would leave the child's legal position in the interval somewhat uncertain.

Another suggestion is that the AID child be adopted. This proposal really comes in two forms: one which suggests that the child be adopted in the usual way, and the other which would involve the child being adopted while it is *in utero*. Adoption is also open to the criticisms mentioned above in connection with the attribution of special status. It would involve disclosure of how the child was conceived, it would take time, and it might result in a legitimate child being adopted by its own father. A couple might also be opposed to adoption if they were in a jurisdiction which allowed access to the birth records. Usually the records of adopted children's natural parents are not open for public inspection, but in the United Kingdom adopted children have the right to ascertain who their natural parents are,[44] because the interests of the child have prevailed over any interests which the natural parents might have in concealing their involvement with adoption. Some have argued that AID children ought to be told about their conception[45] and some would allow them access to a register showing their natural parentage,[46] but donors might be opposed to this. A process which would allow a child to be adopted while it was still *in utero* would require legislative change, and while the couple would not be required to wait for some time *after* the birth before the process was complete, the procedure would have been unnecessary if the child was not born alive or died within a short time of birth. Any procedure undertaken while the child is still *in utero* could not become final at least until its birth.

Another suggestion, which was made by Lord Kilbrandon, is that the register of births be altered to have an entry for 'father or accepting husband'.[47] As has been said, many husbands enter their names as the fathers on the birth records. Such an entry is not conclusive of either paternity or legitimacy, but it would be extremely difficult to prove the contrary. The proposal about acceptance has the merit that it does not involve the couple in inconvenience or embarrassment at the time of registration, but it would require a change in the law on registration of births because it is an offence for a person knowingly to give false information to the registrar. (No doctor should advise his patients to take this course.)

The disadvantage of having an entry for 'father or accepting husband' is that at some later stage the child might wish to know whether the name on the birth certificate was that of his father or the accepting husband, and if it was the latter he might want to know who his 'real' father is. Although Lord Kilbrandon made the suggestion in the context of discussions about the AID child, there is no reason why a husband or wife should not be able to 'accept' any of his or her illegitimate children.

A further suggestion is that the register of births should be concerned only with 'acceptance', and make no mention of 'father'.[48] Where both husband and wife were the biological parents of the child they would be required to register their child as 'accepted' but in all other cases there would be an option. There might be disputes between biological parents and those wishing to 'accept' a child, but these disputes might not be numerous and would be unlikely where the child was an AID child. However a proposal to alter the register of births in this way would have to ensure that people were prevented from 'accepting' any child and so circumventing the adoption legislation.

The notion of 'accepted child' exists already in the case of the child brought up as a member of a family.[49] Such a child is recognized in the UK for the purposes of social security, income tax, maintenance, custody, and aliment,[50] and in England, also for succession.[51] Something akin to 'acceptance' exists in other legal systems in the form of 'acknowledgement' or 'recognition', whereby a man may include within his family a child which he has 'acknowledged' or 'recognized'.[52] It must be admitted however that the acknowledgement or recognition would appear in the register of births and would thus disclose that the child was not a legitimate child. No country has adopted the notion of the 'accepted' child in relation to the AID child, but there are other provisions which deal with the child's status.

'Deeming' provision

The solution which has been most commonly adopted, particularly in the USA, is a statutory provision that where a married woman conceives a child as the result of AID and her husband has consented, the husband is deemed in law to be the father of the child.

Despite many statements to the contrary,[53] the first jurisdiction to introduce this reform was Georgia in 1964. The statute provides:

> All children born within wedlock or within the usual period of gestation thereafter, who have been conceived by the means of artificial insemination, are irrebutably presumed legtitimate if both the husband and the wife consent in writing to the use and administration of artificial insemination.[54]

A similar statute was passed in Oklahoma in 1967[55] and this pattern has been repeated in other states.[56] The principle is now enshrined in the Uniform Parentage Act, section 5(a) of which provides:

> If, under the supervision of a licensed physician and with the consent of her husband, a wife is inseminated artificially with semen donated by a man who is not her husband, the husband is treated in law as if he was the natural father of the child thereby conceived. The husband's consent must be in writing and signed by him and his wife.[57]

Statutory provisions of this kind deal generally with the status of AID children and their legal relationship with the husband and avoid the problems of a more piecemeal approach.

Two points of detail are worthy of mention. The first is that, with the exception of the Kansas statute,[58] the statutory provisions are not retrospective, and so they leave in doubt the status of AID children born prior to the legislation. While this matter has not yet come before a court, judges could decide that the intention of the legislation was to remove the anomalies from all AID children and declare the statutes to be retroactive. This would be a sensible and liberal approach which would result in all AID children being treated in the same way.

The second point is more difficult. Each of the provisions requires that the insemination should be done only with the husband's consent: indeed only the state of Oregon seems to allow artificial insemination for unmarried women.[59] The question which arises is: what is the child's status if that consent has not been given? Several views are possible. One is to say that if the husband does not consent, the child is illegitimate. Alternatively the child will be presumed legitimate because of the marriage, but the non-consenting husband may be able to rebut the presumption; but if he does not he will be regarded as the father. If, however, he does succeed, the status of the child may have to be determined by the courts.

In order to avoid these problems, one writer has suggested that the child should be legitimate whether or not such consent is given. If the consent is not given in writing the onus would be on the wife to establish that the husband gave oral consent. If she could not prove this the husband should be able to divorce his wife on the ground that she had been artificially inseminated without his consent. He justifies his proposal in these terms:

> It is believed that the *father* [sic] has been relieved to a satisfactory degree by granting to him the right to seek divorce. Beyond that he is not protected. This is because the occasion of artificial insemination, without the consent of the husband, where the man and woman are in a state of legal wedlock, is, in most cases, presumably the fault, at least to some degree, of both parties concerned. And it is this majority of situations under which this statute is enacted. Secondly, the state must also be protected, and further protection of the husband would put the greater, if not the whole, burden on the state. Thirdly, and most important, the child, before all others, is to receive the greatest interests of the law. The stigma of illegitimacy can well result in a tragic situation which is to be avoided at all reasonable costs.[60]

The obvious reponse to this suggestion is that it seems strange to saddle a husband with legal responsibility for a child born to his wife where she has been inseminated without his approval. Furthermore there does not seem to be any logical reason why this suggestion should not be applied to a child conceived in adultery.

The statutory provisions emphasize the need for consent and it would be difficult to argue that the absence of consent does not affect the status of the child. It is therefore likely that a court would say that the child is illegitimate if consent is not given.

In order to avoid the difficulties which might arise if the consent form could not be found, there could be a presumption that the husband had given his consent. It would then be up to him to establish that he had not.[61]

Although the main legislative activity in this field has been in the USA, there has been some elsewhere. In Europe there are three jurisdictions which deal with the status of AID children, if only indirectly – Portugal, Switzerland and The Netherlands.[62] The Portuguese Civil Code provides that artificial insemination cannot be invoked to establish or contest the paternity of a child so conceived. The Swiss Civil Code denies a husband any action to disavow paternity of a child if he has consented to its conception through a third party, and the provisions of the Dutch Civil Code are similar. These provisions do not make the AID child legitimate or in an identical position to a legitimate child, which is what the US legislation does; rather they prevent the husband proving that the child is not his legitimate child. In Sweden however legislation makes express provision about the child's status by stating that it shall be regarded for all purposes as the husband's child or the child of the cohabitee, provided in each case that consent was given to the insemination.[63]

In 1979 the Council of Europe produced a Draft Recommendation on Artificial Insemination, Article 7 of which deals with the status of the AID child:[64]

> When artificial insemination has been administered with the consent of the husband, the child shall be considered as the legitimate child of the woman and her husband and nobody may contest the legitimacy on the sole ground of artificial insemination.

A similar approach can be seen in the Private Member's Bill presented to the UK parliament in 1977. That attempt failed and it was not until 1987, with the passing of the Family Law Reform Act 1987, that section 27 introduced a 'deeming' provision for England and Wales. The section has been quoted in full in Chapter 7, but it is worth repeating here, since the importance of the section lies in the fact that it eliminates the most significant anomaly, which is the succession rights of children born as the result of AID. The section, which applies only to England and Wales is as follows:

> Where after the coming into force of this section a child is born in England and Wales as the result of artificial insemination of a woman who

(a) was at the time of the insemination a party to a dissolved or annulled marriage and

(b) was artificially inseminated with the semen of some person other than the other party to that marriage, then, unless it is proved to the satisfaction of any court by which the matter has to be determined that the other party to that marriage did not consent to the insemination, the child shall be treated in law as the child of the parties to that marriage and shall not be treated as the child of any person other than the parties to that marriage.

As has been noted earlier, it does not apply to children born in Scotland, nor does it extend to children born following egg or embryo donation. Like most of the legislation in the USA, it is not retrospective and it applies only where consent has been given. Presumably, when the government Bill, following on the recent White Paper, is introduced, it will extend the Bill to Scotland and also to the other forms of artificial conception.

Although the form of words used in the European countries and in the Draft Recommendation of the Council of Europe differ from each other, and from the US provisions, they have this much in common: they expressly, or by implication, deem the husband to be the father of a child conceived by artificial insemination.

That solution, like that of the 'accepted child', avoids the criticisms levelled against the other solutions, that they might involve a legal process which in some cases would be unnecessary, or that they might cause delay and possibly embarrassment to the couple.

However, both the 'accepted child' notion and the 'deeming' provision are open to the criticism that each conceals the child's true origins both from the child and from society. The 'accepted child' notion would deceive every child, whereas the 'deeming' provision would deceive only AID children, but both would deceive society, in that the register of births would not disclose the child's true paternity. The question whether there ought to be this concealment or not is dealt with later, but it is appropriate to say something about it here.

With the 'deeming' provision, the birth register would be inaccurate unless there was another register showing 'true' origins. If such a register existed it would have to be determined who should have access to it and in what circumstances. Presumably, on the analogy of adoption, only someone who could show good cause – and this will usually be only the adopted child – should have access.

The creation of a register of true origins also involves donors who would have to be advised that, at some later stage, the children would be able to identify them. To what extent donors would continue to be willing to participate in AID programmes if this were the case is a matter of conjecture. A 'half-way house' solution might be to have a register giving certain relevant particulars about the donor, principally medical and genetic information, without disclosing his actual identity.

While the question of whether any kind of second register ought to be kept is important, it is more important to resolve the status of the AID child. The solution adopted must recognize that the child is a member of the husband's family and not of any other, but couples must be able to go through the process without undue delay or special, and possibly lengthy, procedures and it should not involve them in embarrassment. The 'deeming' provision satisfies all these requirements and it is suggested that this should be introduced into Scots law without further delay, and be extended to egg and embryo donation.

9 Confidentiality and disclosure

In this chapter two separate but related issues are examined. The first is whether the doctor is under an obligation to disclose the involvement of his patients and donors in AID; and the second is whether the child ought to be told of the circumstances of its conception, and whether information about the donor should be made available to the child and/or the 'parents'. The issues are related because disclosure by the doctor might provide the child with some knowledge about its conception and also give the mother some information about the donor. The first question is looked at under the heading 'Confidentiality' and the second under 'Disclosure'. Clearly there is no reason why a doctor should not admit that he provides an AID service, and so this chapter is concerned only with disclosure about patients and donors. As with other aspects of AID, the principles apply equally to egg donation and embryo donation, and for convenience 'AID' and 'donor' cover all three.

Confidentiality

There are a number of points which can be raised here. The doctor's general ethical code[1] may give some guidance in relation to disclosure of information about AID. Whether or not this guidance exists, it is important to ask whether there is a *legal* obligation to disclose or not to disclose such details. The last point is whether, assuming that the doctor is required by his ethical code or by law *not* to disclose these details, there are circumstances in which disclosure would nevertheless be justified.

Ethical codes

It is rather misleading to talk of *an* ethical code which regulates the doctor's approach to the subject of confidentiality, in that there are several ethical declarations which deal with disclosure of information. These range from universal codes, such as the Hippocratic Oath and the International Code of Ethics of the World Medical Association, to codes which apply to the medical profession in one country, such as those of the British and American Medical Associations.[2]

It is outside the scope of this book to embark upon a detailed examination of these codes, but it is important to note that there are major differences between them. For example, the Declaration of Geneva (1948) is in absolute terms: 'I will hold in confidence all that my patient confides in me'; whereas the Principles of Medical Ethics of the American Medical Association (1971) list three exceptions to the rule that 'a physician may not reveal the confidences entrusted in him in the course of medical attendance'. These exceptions are:

(a)   when the doctor is required by law to make a disclosure of confidential information;
(b)   when such a disclosure is necessary to protect the welfare of the individual or of the society;
(c)   when the disclosure is authorized by the patient.

Clearly if a code is expressed in absolute terms, then any disclosure of confidential information would be a breach. Such a code would require a doctor not to reveal information about the donors or recipients, but as we have noted, the Principles of Medical Ethics of the AMA are not expressed in such absolute terms.

Many AID couples and donors would probably not authorize the doctor to reveal information about them, and it is unlikely that the doctor would be able to justify disclosure on the basis that it was in the interests of either the individuals or society. The only situation which would justify disclosure is when there is a legal obligation to reveal information, which will be dealt with shortly.

While these ethical formulae are important, it is not possible to say whether the majority of doctors are aware of their terms nor to what extent they regard confidentiality as being governed by them. The doctor's approach to the subject may be dictated by purely practical considerations, which should not be underestimated. To make a correct diagnosis and prescribe appropriate treatment, the doctor must have complete and accurate information about the patient. He is unlikely to obtain this unless the patient feels that he can be completely frank with the doctor, and he will feel that way only if he knows that what the doctor finds out about him will be treated in confidence.

In relation to AI, this is of particular importance. Before a doctor will prescribe AI, he will have to obtain from the couple intimate details of their sex lives and they will not be forthcoming about these unless they are certain that this information will not be disclosed.

Confidentiality is also an important element in the doctor/donor relationship. The doctor will wish to preserve anonymity about the donor to encourage him to become and remain a donor; otherwise persons might be deterred from being donors. In addition if the donor knows that the doctor will not reveal information about him he will feel more free to discuss his medical and family history, and during such a discussion the doctor might discover something which suggests that a particular donor should not be used. The donor might wish to know about this, but he would not necessarily wish others to be told.

Legal duty not to disclose

There are three senses in which there may be a legal obligation on the doctor not to disclose confidential information. First, disclosure may be prohibited by statute. The New York City Health Code[3] and legislation in two states in Yugoslavia[4] expressly prohibit the disclosure of information about AID. Some of the United States legislation provides for filing information about AID with the state authorities,[5] who have the sole right to determine who shall have access to it. By implication the doctor is required to keep his involvement secret, but in none of this legislation is there mention of any penalty for failure to comply with the provisions. Secondly unauthorized disclosure could result either in the doctor's suspension from practice or the removal of his name from the list of those entitled to practise.[6] This might be a consequence of an unauthorized disclosure under the legislation just mentioned.

In the UK such disclosure may amount to 'serious professional misconduct',[7] and occasionally the professional bodies have had to consider such cases, although not in relation to AID.[8] In the USA the corresponding term is 'malpractice', and many courts have held that unauthorized disclosure amounts to malpractice, at least for insurance purposes, but again this has not arisen in connection with AID.[9] In Michigan, for example, unauthorized disclosure is a criminal offence[10] and some countries in Europe[11] and elsewhere[12] have similar provisions in their criminal codes.

Even if the prohibition is not expressed in such general terms the doctor may be required by statute not to disclose details of his treatment of certain conditions, for example venereal disease.[13] This too is a matter for the criminal law.

The final sense in which there may be an obligation to respect the patient's confidence is that the courts will prevent a threatened unauthorized disclosure, or give an award of damages if such a disclosure is made. These remedies lie within the province of the civil, and not the criminal, law. The relationship between the doctor and his patient may be contractual, as in the USA,[14] and there may be an implied term in the contract that the doctor will treat as confidential all that the patient tells him and everything which he ascertains as the result of examining the patient. If the doctor threatens to reveal information, the patient may take steps to prevent that, because the doctor's conduct would amount to breach of contract. If the doctor does disclose confidential details, that would be a breach of contract for which the courts would award damages.[15] That would also be the case where a patient in the UK consulted a doctor outside the NHS.

However there are also rights and duties which do not depend upon the existence of a contract between the parties. These arise by virtue of the law of delict/tort,[16] and a person who has suffered loss as the result of the wrongful disclosure of confidential information may sue whether there is a contract with the doctor or not. In the UK the patient will not have a contract with his doctor under the NHS[17] but he could sue in delict/tort. The courts could be asked to prevent a threatened unauthorized disclosure or give damages where such a disclosure has been made. In this area however the law in the UK is less well-developed than in the USA.

England   In England the courts have only recently begun to recognize breach of confidence as a separate tort. In the nineteenth century there were a number of judicial observations to the effect that a doctor was not in a privileged position in court proceedings, which thereby allowed him to withhold information about his patient. Little guidance was available on whether there was a legal obligation not to breach the patient's confidence. One case which is frequently cited for the existence of such an obligation is *Kitson v. Playfair*,[18] but that action was based on slander, in other words it was alleged that what the doctor had said was false and derogatory of the plaintiff. However, although the case was not based on breach of confidence, the judge did assume that a medical practitioner was under a legal duty not to make unauthorized disclosure of information about his patients. More recently Lord Denning said that a court would respect professional confidence and would not require a person to breach that, 'unless not only it is relevant but also it is a proper and, indeed, a necessary question in the course of justice to be put and answered.'[19] However that observation was made in a case where journalists had refused to reveal sources of information and was not concerned with the more general issue of breach of confidence, nor specifically with doctors.

But in *Seager v. Copydex Limited*[20] breach of confidence was in issue and while the case did not deal with doctors general comments were made, again by Lord Denning:

> The law on this subject does not depend on any implied contract. It depends on the broad principle of equity that he who has received information in confidence shall not take unfair advantage of it. He must not make use of it to the prejudice of him who gave it without obtaining his consent.

Scotland   In Scotland the courts recognized the obligation to respect confidence at a much earlier stage. In a case in 1851[21] the pursuer was a church elder whose wife had given birth to a child within six months of their marriage. The minister requested 'respectable medical testimony' to ascertain whether the child had been conceived before or after the marriage. The doctor was asked to make the necessary examination, and he concluded that the child had been conceived before the marriage. The doctor wrote his report and a copy was left for the minister. The elder was removed from office and he brought a successful action against the doctor for breach of confidence. As one of the judges said: 'The question here is, not whether the communications of a medical adviser are privileged – that cannot be maintained; but whether the relationship between such an adviser and the person who consults him, is or is not one which may imply an obligation to secrecy, forming a proper ground of action if it be violated.' In another case, decided in 1904,[22] the same view was taken. Both the Law Commission and the Scottish Law Commission[23] have recommended that breach of confidence be recognized by statute as an actionable wrong, but no legislation has, as yet, followed.

USA[24]   In the USA greater consideration has been given to the legal issues surrounding the doctor/patient relationship than in the UK. In the USA that relationship receives protection in two ways; one is based on statute law; the other on common law, that is, judicial decision. The statutory protection is known as 'privileged communication', whereas the common law doctrine is that of 'confidential communications'.[25] These notions are distinct. The object of the statutory provisions on privileged communication is to prevent disclosure in court of confidential information. If the doctor breaches that obligation he may be prohibited from practising, since such conduct is regarded as malpractice. The common law on confidential communications is intended to prevent a doctor from disclosing confidential information in all other circumstances. If the doctor is in breach of that obligation he may be liable for damages for breach of confidence.

As a general rule a doctor would not be permitted to disclose his professional involvement with a patient to any third party. Applying that to AID, a doctor should not reveal to anyone the fact that a woman has requested or received AID, far less that she has given birth to a child as a result. The law in the USA and the UK on this point is therefore similar.

Legally justifiable disclosure

The next point is whether there are any circumstances in which a doctor will be protected if he does disclose information which would normally be considered confidential. The privileges which have been mentioned are not absolute,[26] because there are a number of situations in which disclosure is permitted – for example where the patient has given prior consent to the disclosure or where a third party has an overriding need for the information. The welfare of the patient or the need to protect society may also justify disclosure, as will a statute or a court order. It is necessary for present purposes to examine each of these exceptions only briefly.

Where the patient has given consent to the disclosure of confidential information the doctor is clearly protected, but it is unlikely that a patient undergoing AID would give such consent or that a third party (apart possibly from the AID child) could demonstrate a need for the information. Some people have argued that the child has a right to know his origins and the corollary of that is that if the child asked, the doctor should tell him about AID. This has never been discussed, but the doctor's ethics and perhaps the law would prevent him from disclosing his patient's involvement with AID. Some cases which have raised this matter have permitted disclosure where it fulfils a moral or social duty, provided the information is given in good faith and is not in disregard of the patient's wishes.[27] It is possible to use as an analogy adoption cases in which the adopted child is seeking information about its natural parents.[28] While there are similarities between adopted children and AID children, special provision has been made for adopted children in the UK whereas none exists for AID children.[29] Until it does, it would not be safe for a doctor to disclose information to the child unless required by a court to do so.

Other factors are the welfare of the patient and the interests of society. It is difficult to think of a situation in which it would be in the patient's interests for the doctor to disclose that she had been given AID and it seems unlikely that an argument based on society's needs would be successful. This matter is more fully explored later in the discussion of 'disclosure'.

The final situation in which a doctor would be permitted to

disclose information about his patient's involvement with AID would be where a statute required this. The only statutes which deal with disclosure of AID are those in the USA, but, as has been said, they require the doctor to disclose information about AID only to the state authority and it is clear that all other disclosures would be unauthorized.Other provisions which require doctors to disclose information deal with such matters as communicable diseases, as there may be a very real threat to members of the public if information is not available.

In conclusion therefore, there is nothing, apart from a court order, which would justify a disclosure by a doctor about AID, and a court is likely to make such an order only where the information is central to the proper conduct of a litigation. Up till now, litigation in respect of AID has been rare and, as far as we can trace, there is no case in which a doctor has been required to reveal that he provided AID to one of the litigants.

Disclosure

The obligations which may govern the doctor's conduct obviously cannot dictate how patients should act. However there is little publicity about AID and it seems that the majority of couples are not in favour of disclosing that they have had AID, and that many couples do not tell the children about how they were conceived.

In this section there are three separate but related issues. One is whether the public or the state ought to know which children have been conceived by AID; another is whether the identity of the donor ought to be revealed; and the third is whether the child ought to be told about the circumstances of his conception, and perhaps also be able to find out who the donor was. The issues are separate in that the reasons which can be put forward for not making information about AID children public may not be valid reasons for keeping the donor's identity secret or for not telling the child. They are related in that any disclosure to the child might result in his origins being more widely known, and any disclosure of a public nature, for example in the birth registers, can become known to the child. If the identity of the donor is revealed to the child, that may also result in the child's identity being made known to the donor.

The interests of the various parties (apart from the doctor) – the AID couple, the donor as the biological parent, the child and the public or the state – must be considered but two preliminary points should be made. The first is that these various interests may conflict. The second is that there are no reported cases on these issues, but some of the US statutes are relevant. However, because there are certain similarities between AID children and adopted children, some assistance may be had from legislation and case law in that field.

The AID couple

There are two main reasons why a couple may not wish it to be known that the woman has undergone AID; their union may be infertile, or it may not be advisable for the man to father children. It can be argued that, if people have the psychological trauma of infertility or are likely to pass on some deleterious condition to their children, the less they are reminded of it the better.

There may also be a social stigma attaching to those who have to resort to artificial insemination, just as there may be for those who adopt a child. In this connection, the man may be especially vulnerable in that he might feel that his sense of parenthood is being threatened.

The next point is whether the identity of the donor ought to be revealed to the couple. At present the doctor would not be permitted to make disclosure, and if such disclosures were made that might dissuade people from becoming donors. Another consideration which might concern the husband is the possibility that his wife's affection might be diverted from him to the donor. There is evidence that women who receive AID have 'a strong need to dissociate from thought and concern about the meaning of the donor to them'.[30] If the risk of some psychological longing for the donor does exist, it might be intensified if his identity became known.

If the donor's identity is to be revealed to the couple, the corollary is whether their identity should be revealed to him. It is tempting to argue that the one disclosure is a counterpart of the other, but there are separate arguments for not disclosing the identity of the couple. They might be concerned that this would result in the donor interfering in the child's upbringing. He might, for example, make suggestions about the child's education or religion or make a claim should the child die leaving a large estate. The couple's concern might be that such interference would prevent or hinder the formation and development of a stable relationship between them and the child.

If the couple knew the identity of the donor they would have to decide whether or not to tell the child about him. There are really two questions here. One is whether to tell the child in general terms about AID, which would not make the donor's identity known. The second is whether they should tell the child who the donor is, or was.

The couple might not wish to say anything about AID to the child because they would find it difficult or embarrassing to do so. They might also feel that it might upset the child to be told that the person or persons whom he regards as his father and/or mother is, or are, not his biological parent or parents.

If they did decide to tell the child about the AID they might still not wish to reveal the donor's identity, even if they knew it. They could argue that the child should not be informed because he will always regard the husband or male partner as his father. If the child is told who the donor was, he would then be in the position of having two fathers or mothers or both. That might result in divided loyalty and have an adverse effect on the child.

There is some support for that approach, in that there is a school of thought which holds that what is important for a child is not that he is aware of his biological origins, but that he has social or psychological parents and is brought up in a family unit.[31] On that view it is not necessary to tell the child even about his conception.

The last, but very important, reason why a couple may wish to maintain this secrecy is that in many jurisdictions the child in this situation is considered illegitimate, or its legal status is uncertain. Even in the USA, where there is legislation, only in Kansas is it retrospective.[32] In the other states the status of the child conceived or born prior to the passing of the relevant statute remains in doubt. While it must be admitted that there is less discrimination against illegitimate children than formerly, they still do not always occupy the same position in law or society as legitimate children. For these reasons the couple will not wish the child to be regarded as illegitimate, or run the risk that it may be declared so by the courts. Birth entries are frequently falsified to eliminate these possibilities.

Having outlined the reasons for not disclosing details about AID, there may be situations in which the couple will want information about the donor, or may wish to tell the child about his conception.

One of the concerns of adopting parents is whether the child has inherited any characteristics from his natural parents which might adversely affect his health or development. Some concern is also felt over behaviour and personality problems.[33] These may concern the 'parents' of AID children, but concern may be less acute, since in this situation one parent is biologically related to the child. It might however arise in embryo donation where neither 'parent' has a biological tie. Even if this concern exists, it is not a reason for disclosing the *identity* of the donor to the couple but merely for disclosing sufficient information to give the couple guidance.

However in most, if not all, instances couples seeking AID will be given some details or assurances about the donor. For example, in the explanatory booklet produced by the RCOG the following statement is made:

> The donors are carefully selected. They are required to be intelligent, fit and healthy and in questioning to have given no family history of hereditary disease. They must all be of very high fertility and every specimen of semen is checked before it is used to make sure that it reaches an acceptable standard.

Similar guidance is given in the New York City Health Code which requires that a sperm donor be free from venereal disease, tuberculosis, brucellosis and any congenital disease. These requirements are discussed more fully in Chapter 10.

Disclosure of details about the donor would not invade his privacy, but what the couple are told at interview may be as much information as is available, and that perhaps satisfies most, if not all, couples.

Although the couple may not wish to know who the donor was, or even to know much about him, there are occasions when they may want to tell the child how he was conceived, for example where the reason for undergoing AID is that the man suffers or may suffer from some condition which makes it undesirable for him to father children. One example of this is Huntington's Chorea, where an afflicted person has a 50 per cent chance of passing the condition on to his offspring. If the couple therefore decide to undergo AID because the man suffers, or could suffer, from Huntington's Chorea, they may wish to tell the child that he has been conceived by AID, in order to reassure him that he is not afflicted in the same way as his 'father'.

The donor

Having examined the interests of the couple, we now consider those of the donor. There does not seem to be any reason why a donor would wish his identity to be revealed to the child or the couple, but he might not object to some other details about him being given to them. Like the couple, the donor may wish to protect himself against any stigma which could attach to his involvement with AID. In addition he may wish to avoid embarrassment, or disruption of his private life, which might be caused by the appearance of a child whose existence may be unknown to his spouse or partner. There might, for example, be a claim by the child for maintenance or, more seriously, a claim by the child on the donor's estate after his death. Donor semen may have been used on more than one occasion, and so, numerous claims could be made. That could mean that his estate would be diminished considerably and it would not be possible to wind it up until all potential claims had been identified.

In any event the donor will probably have been assured by the doctor that his identity will not be revealed. If such an assurance has been given, the donor is entitled to rely on it.

The child

As we have seen, there are a number of reasons why couples and donors would wish their involvement with AID to be kept secret. We must now consider the interests of the child, and in particular whether the child should know the identity of, or details about, the donor.

In the context of adoption, the recommendation is that the child should be told about it, and at an early age.[34] The reason given for this advice is that it can be psychologically disturbing for an adopted child not to know who his natural parents were. The consequences of not knowing can be insecurity and an under-developed sense of identity.[35] This school of thought has influenced the UK parliament and some legislatures and judges in the USA and elsewhere, for example Sweden. We shall therefore look at the developments in the area of adoption law and then consider the extent to which these can or should be applied to AID.

In Scotland an adopted child who is seventeen, and in England eighteen, may inspect the registers to try to identify his natural parents.[36] The Registrar-General is required to keep records which will enable adopted children to make the necessary connection between the entry in the Adopted Children's Register and the original birth entry. These records are not available for public inspection, but if an adopted child wishes to go through this exercise there are counselling facilities available to him.[37]

In the USA the position is less clear. While most states have legislation dealing with disclosure,[38] there is considerable doubt about which states permit an adopted child to obtain a copy of his original birth certificate or court records about the adoption.[39] There are 'open' statutes and 'closed' statutes. One type of open statute permits the adopted child to have access to the records once he has reached the age of majority,[40] but in only one state, Virginia, is access permitted to the court records.[41] In most states the records are 'closed' and disclosure is generally not permitted.[42] Nevertheless even in those states there is usually an exception where the applicant can show 'good cause'.[43] In recent court cases there has been a trend in favour of taking into account the psychological needs of the adopted child, but the approach of the courts, not surprisingly, has varied. In the case of *In re Ann Carol S*,[44] a New York court permitted an adult who had been adopted to have access to her birth records. She had shown that she had been obsessed by a need to obtain this information. The Supreme Court of New Jersey considered the issue in *Lovallo v. NJ State Registrar*.[45] The court held that an adoptee's psychological need to know the identity of the biological parents might constitute 'good cause', and it laid down guidelines for dealing with such requests by adopted persons. In the case of adults seeking such details, the court said that it was for the state to demonstrate that good cause did not exist. In every case however the court had to be satisfied that a procedure existed for protecting the interests of the biological parents, under the Equal Protection provisions in the Constitution. Traditionally there had to be a rational basis for the discrimination in relation to the purpose of the statute.[46] More recently the courts have required the classification to have a 'fair and substantial relation to the object of the legislation'.[47] The adopted person might experience difficulty in establishing that there was no rational basis for discrimination in relation to the non-disclosure of information. Under the more recent test he would have to show that the purpose of the legislation was to further the interests of adopted persons, and that might be equally difficult.

However, even if the adopted person's arguments were persuasive, they would have to be considered along with the reasons for non-disclosure. It could be suggested that the records are sealed to protect the privacy of the biological parents and that the public interest demands that the adoption process be kept out of the glare of publicity so far as is possible. Another point is that the adopted person would have to show that the disclosure would be beneficial for the majority of adoptees and not just for the person who was petitioning for it.

An alternative approach, but one which is still based on equal protection, is to argue that the statutes which require adoption records to be kept secret create a 'suspect classification', or that they compromise a 'fundamental right'. Statutes which come into this category have been subjected to much closer scrutiny, and are presumed invalid unless they further some significant state interest. A 'suspect classification' was defined by the US Supreme Court in 1973 to be 'an immutable characteristic determined solely by birth'.[48] Illegitimacy has been recognized as similar to such a characteristic,[49] but not all adopted children are illegitimate and neither are the children conceived as the result of AID. The statutory provisions in some states deem such children to be legitimate, and so it would seem that AID children are not a 'suspect class'. On the assumption that this approach is not open, the second strand of the argument is that a person's identity is a 'fundamental right', and it can be argued that there is nothing more fundamental than one's identity. No matter how forceful these points might seem, the adopted person must persuade the court on one further point, namely that the interests which are protected by the state are not 'compelling'. This point will be developed when considering the public or state interest.

Some statutes require doctors to file certain information about AID births with the state authorities, but they provide that the records are available for inspection only if a court order has been granted 'on cause [or good] cause' shown. While the matter has never arisen, one can assume that the file may be made available to the child on cause shown, but it might not be enough to show that the child was an AID child. The cause, or good cause, would probably still have to be established.

Not all states have such legislation but because there are undoubtedly similarities between AID children and adopted children, it could be argued that what has been done for adopted children ought to be done also for AID children. However there are also significant differences which should be noted before a conclusion is reached on whether an AID child ought to have access to such information.

Reasons for not disclosing details about AID

It is probably essential to tell the adopted child about the adoption, where the adoptive mother is not also the natural mother. If the adoptive parents do not say anything about the adoption prior to the child's arrival in their home, the fact that the woman has not been pregnant will inevitably prompt relatives, neighbours and friends to inquire about the child's origins. Once they know, the child will inevitably find out, even by inadvertence. Accordingly it is better that the child should be told by the parents, rather than by someone else. In the case of the child conceived by AID, because the woman will have been pregnant, there is nothing which suggests that the child is not the couple's child.

It might be observed however that some adopted children have a psychological need to know about their origins. It is not enough to point to the psychological need felt by some adopted children, without going further and demonstrating that there is also a need in the case of AID children. The psychological need in adopted children possibly arises because they are aware that the adoptive parents are not their natural parents. The question is whether AID children, or indeed adopted children, would have this need if they were not told about the adoption or the artificial insemination.

The second point is that, while official records of the birth of an adopted child do exist, no similar records exist about the conception of AID children. In their case the doctors may *have* records, but they are not official nor will they prove conclusively who the parents are. These records are not usually made available by doctors and they are not obliged to disclose what is in them. Accordingly a couple who wished to tell their child about his conception would not be able to say who the child's father was. That being so, it might be more harmful to give the child only this limited amount of information than it would be not to mention AID at all, except where it is undertaken to avoid an inheritable disorder being transmitted to the child. Where information about an AID child is lodged with a state authority, both the couple and the child would probably be able to obtain access if they could show cause, or good cause.

Reasons for disclosing details about AID

There are two main arguments in favour of disclosure. One is the risk of a consanguineous marriage sometimes called 'incest', and the other is that the child has a 'right' to know.

Consanguineous marriage Making the child aware of its origins should avoid an unwitting marriage between offspring of the same donor, or between the donor and his daughter or an egg donor and her son. The possibility of an unwitting marriage between offspring of the same donor is something which concerns some AID couples. This must be distinguished from 'incest' which is the crime of having sexual intercourse with someone who is known to be within the prohibited degree of relationship. The marriage of such persons is a matter for the civil law, and many jurisdictions declare such marriages to be void, whether or not the parties were aware that they were prohibited from marrying.

Two comments which have been made on this subject are instructive: 'The incest taboo is one of the strongest in our society. There can be little doubt that the increasing production of children by means of artificial insemination from unknown donors enhances the possibilities of incestuous marriages and incestuous relationships.'[50] The following observation is of a similar nature:

> The chances of a man unknowingly marrying a woman artificially conceived with his own seed are perhaps rather slight. But much more likely is the possibility of marriage between persons conceived with semen from the same donor, especially where the doctors keep 'sperm banks' and dilute the sperm to such an extent that a great number of conceptions can be effected from a single ejaculation.[51]

The difficulty about such statements is that they do not give any indication of how great the risk is, but on a fair reading they give the impression that it is significant. However they do not cite any literature in support of the views expressed.

When the subject was investigated by the Feversham Committee in 1958–60, it was concluded that the danger of a marriage between children of the same donor was 'at present minimal'. The committee was informed by the late Professor D. V. Glass, Professor of Sociology in the University of London, that if 2000 live children were born in Great Britain as the result of AID and if each donor was responsible for five children, 'an unwitting incestuous marriage is unlikely to occur more than once in about fifty to a hundred years. Thus even if there were a twenty-fold increase in the use of AID, as compared with our estimate of its present incidence, the possibility that two children having the same father would marry would be remote.'[52] Two more recent reports confirm this view.[53] The Feversham Report, however, continues on a cautionary note: 'although if a much wider use were made of each donor and if practitioners drew their patients from small areas, the possibility would increase'.[54] Any argument for telling the child that is based on the risk of incest or consanguineous marriage is therefore of little weight.

The right to know   The second argument is that the child has a 'right' to know about its origins. This 'right' is different from the notion of moral rights which impose a corresponding duty and it differs also from ethical principles which are expressed in more general terms. Even if a person has a 'right' to know, the information may not be available. Many illegitimate children will not be able to find out who their fathers are. An AID child is in no worse position than these children in this respect, but of course may be better off in others.

A much sounder argument is that it is wrong to deceive the child about its origins. This is a powerful argument and one which is difficult to refute.

However, the 'right to know' argument, and the argument based on 'deception', if accepted, would come into conflict with other people's interests and wishes, the most obvious examples being the couple and the donor. In coming to any conclusion about this, one would have to balance the harm caused to the child by not knowing about his origins against the desire of the couple to keep intimate details of the marriage a secret, and the risk that people may be dissuaded from being donors if there is a risk that their identities may be revealed. This is clearly a matter on which any legislature would seek a number of views and any decision would have to take into account the interests of the state itself.

The public or state interest

It is often argued that society should be able to identify children
with their parents and that if the register of births is falsified,
then society is deceived. However when the Feversham Committee
looked at this issue they doubted whether society had such a right,
and gave two reasons for this view. The first was that in most of
our dealings with other people it is generally of no consequence to
know who their parents are. The second was that a society which
permits a person to use any name he wishes can hardly claim to be
anxious to ascertain a person's origins. Nevertheless the committee
acknowledged that the practice of AID does involve 'the permanent
deception of a considerable number of people'.[55]

While there may be some force in the committee's view, there
are groups within society who have a legitimate interest in the
accuracy of birth records. For example, historians and those
working with titles of honour can make useful comment only if
they can be sure that the records they are examining are accurate;
and those involved in genetics and genetic counselling are
completely dependent upon knowing the truth about biological
parentage. Moreover as a general proposition it might be said that
society has, or should have, an interest in seeking truth for its own
sake, and so it is desirable that its records be as accurate as possible.
Further, if AID is carried out in secret it is not possible to conduct
a critical examination of the practice and its consequences.[56] It is
frequently the case that the medical practitioner is solely responsible
for the processes of interviewing and counselling the couples,
selecting the donors and delivering the children. Any follow-up
studies of couples or children would involve skills other than purely
medical, and more persons would then become aware of the
couples, the children and their involvement with AID.

There are several arguments against disclosure, some of which
relate to privacy. The state may wish to ensure that the AID service
continues and it might be thought that, if the identities of donors
were revealed, this would prejudice the continuance of the service.
It might also wish to discourage claims being made through its
courts on the estate of donors by children seeking maintenance or
a share of estates. The state might also wish to protect the couple
and their children from any stigma which could result from
disclosure of the origins of the child. It might regard the disclosure
of the identity of the donor as a potential threat to the stability of
the AID family.

Conclusion

Several things can be stated clearly. Ethical codes which govern medical practice or an individual doctor's ethical viewpoint would not permit him to disclose anything more than a general involvement with AID and how he practises it. In other words he may talk generally about AID, but must not identify the couples or his donors or the children, unless required by law to do so.

Secondly, although some statutory provisions in the US require doctors to file specific information about AID, they do not permit him to make any other disclosures apart from the general ones just mentioned. It is probably not desirable to make any changes to these rules and principles.

When one turns to the others involved, there are no generally recognized ethical codes, legislation or case law to govern their conduct. A couple who undergo AID will obviously want some information about donors in general and perhaps about the donor who was used, and in all probability they will be given this information. After the child is born, they may continue to wonder who the donor was, but as the child grows up they will gradually concentrate their attention on it and perhaps, in time, forget about the donor. The more they recall the donor, the more they are reminded of the reasons for undergoing AID. They may wish to forget, and will probably not want to tell others. Clearly legislation could not require couples to tell their child if they did not wish to do so. All that legislation can do is require doctors to disclose information and perhaps make that information available to the couples and/or the children. At present doctors are not required to register this information and it is obvious that birth registers are falsified, for whatever reason. It would be foolish to believe that this happens only with AID, but there is an argument that it should not happen deliberately.

The central issue however is whether the child ought to be told. In some cases it will be desirable to tell the child. It may be impossible to avoid telling it where the husband might have passed some disorder on to his children. Where AID is undertaken because the husband is infertile it is necessary to balance the advantages and disadvantages of telling the child against the interests of others. Although some studies have been undertaken on AID,[57] much more could be done. It is interesting to note that in Sweden an AID child has the right at the age of eighteen to find out who its natural father was.[58] The government committee which proposed this was influenced by studies on adopted persons which has been carried out in the USA, the UK and elsewhere.[59]

Egg donation and embryo donation

What has been said about confidentiality in relation to AID applies equally to egg donation and embryo donation. The various interests noted under the heading 'disclosure' exist also in cases of egg and embryo donation and the same arguments for and against telling the child are applicable.

10 Recruitment, selection and matching of donors

The success of any AID service depends primarily on two things – one is the availability of suitable donors and the other is the selection of suitable recipients. The principles behind recruitment etc. for AID apply also to egg donation and embryo donation.

There are however several practical problems. One that is of immediate concern to the couple is the risk that the child will be affected by some disease or disability. (Perhaps all that a couple contemplating AID can expect is that the risk to the child should be no greater than if the husband was the father.)

Another point concerns society, which becomes involved if things go wrong. A society will wish to ensure that the risks of any children born as the result of AID being mentally or physically handicapped or disadvantaged in some other way, or of an unwitting marriage between a child and the donor or between children of the same donor, are as low as possible. The final point is that society has an interest in who are selected as 'parents' for AID to ensure that they are no less suitable for parenthood than other sectors of society, and that there is no deliberate attempt to create 'superior' individuals as there was in the Third Reich. These factors ought to be borne in mind when both donors and couples are being selected.

Donors

The Feversham Committee noted in 1960 that it was extremely difficult to find suitable persons to act as donors.[1] The shortage of donors was also mentioned by some writers at the time,[2] and many doctors still face this problem.[3] But whether or not there is a scarcity of suitable donors it is right to consider what ought to be the criteria for recruitment, selection and matching. There are two main reasons for this. One is that those who are involved in recruiting and so on will, it is hoped, wish to achieve the highest standards.

The second is the related legal issue that those who do the recruiting and so on may subject themselves to liability if they fail to maintain these standards.

In this chapter 'recruitment' means the way in which persons are informed about AID and are asked to volunteer as donors. 'Selection' is the process by which those who are for some reason unsuitable as donors are excluded from those who have been recruited, and 'matching' means the choice of a particular donor for a particular couple.

Very little has been written about recruitment, selection and matching of egg and embryo donors. Some of the detail which follows is obviously not applicable, but the general rules should be.

Recruitment

Who should be donors?   Many practitioners select AID donors from among medical students and house doctors. Perhaps they will also include the husbands of patients, but all these persons have one thing in common – that is, that they are personally known to the doctor. The practice of using medical students seems to have the approval of a majority of authors who have recently written on the subject,[4] and in the past some have declared a preference for students.[5] One writer in the UK has recruited seventy medical students, not one of whom was sterile.[6] In Canada, 80 per cent of donors are students[7] and this is usually the case in Spain.[8] In the USA most doctors (62 per cent) use medical students or hospital residents,[9] but one commentator, writing in 1942, flatly rejected medical students and house doctors and preferred 'physicians and true scientists.'[10]

As the practice of AID expanded, some found it necessary to extend recruiting activities to the public at large.[11] Some have recruited only from among married persons, and this is the position in France since the inauguration of the national CECOS service.[12] In France donors must be under fifty with one or more normal children. Others share this approach. For example the International Planned Parenthood Federation has this to say:

> The donor should have a mature, friendly and cooperative temperament. He must realise that he will never know the children he has fathered and must be mature enough to accept this. Usually he is unable to do so before the age of 25 years, and most doctors do not accept donors over the age of 35. Married donors with children of their own are most stable and are to be desired, since they are unlikely to be promiscuous and open to sexually transmitted infection. Also, their own children show what sort of genetic inheritance the donor is likely to

pass on. It is important to watch out for a history of unwanted recessive genes in the donor's family.[13]

On balance a majority favour using married donors whose fertility has been demonstrated, but much will obviously depend upon the availability of donors. In one person's experience, approaching married donors resulted in only 1 in 10 being recruited.[14] This contrasts markedly with those who have used university students where 95 per cent of those approached agreed to become donors.[15] In Israel the rules issued by the Ministry of Health prohibit the use of donors who are married.[16]

Who should be recruited and by whom? Another question about recruitment concerns those who are doing the recruiting, and who they recruit. Widely-differing views are held about who should be recruited, but, as has been noted, many doctors seem to recruit from among medical students or hospital residents. Sociobiologists would have predicted that. In his book *The Selfish Gene*[17] Richard Dawkins has this to say: 'Ideally what an individual would "like" (I don't mean physically enjoy, although he might) would be to copulate with as many members of the opposite sex as possible, leaving the partner in each case to bring up the children.' It could be argued that by recruiting intending members of the medical profession to be donors, doctors are making a judgment that society would benefit from the 'superior' qualities which members of the medical profession have. More realistically however medical students are readily available.

If doctors tend to select medical students for their 'superior' qualities, and that is objectionable, the objection could be got round, in part at least, by doctors widening their criteria of suitability, but that still leaves the criticism that it is the doctor who makes the selection. That could be overcome if the recruitment and selection were done by a panel with representatives of a number of disciplines, for example psychologists, sociologists, clergymen and doctors. Doctors may find such a procedure cumbersome, but it must be open to doubt whether they themselves have the necessary training, or the authority of society, to select 'suitable' parents for a child. If the analogy of adoption is considered, the state oversees its operation and it has not empowered doctors to make decisions about who are suitable parents. Doctors of course might respond by saying that there is no evidence to support either view that those currently involved in selecting prospective adopters are any better than doctors, or that doctors would be a less satisfactory body than those currently involved.

Payment   This subject was mentioned by the Feversham Committee but not discussed. It was noted that some doctors paid the donor a fee, usually to cover travelling expenses; others made no payment. One witness suggested to the committee that if a payment was made it would put the practice on a more objective basis and would relieve the doctor of having to rely on personal contacts to recruit donors. The committee observed: 'The fact that in this country donors have not been paid for their services has, we understand, had the effect of excluding from the field undesirable persons.'[18]

Some practitioners still do not pay their donors. When the French system, CECOS, was being set up, it was thought that the selling of semen could lead to the abuses which bedevilled the donation of blood in the United States. Those responsible for CECOS were not convinced that offering payments generated a greater interest from donors. Indeed they thought that some potential donors might regard any involvement as morally less attractive if a payment was made, and it might also result in the public becoming disinterested.[19] It would be rather difficult to ascertain whether undesirable persons were dissuaded from being donors because they would not be paid, or whether payment might dissuade desirable donors from participating.

The principle that donors should not be paid was accepted by the Council of Europe in their Draft Recommendation on Artificial Insemination of Human Beings, which has been approved by the European Committees on Legal Cooperation (CDCJ) and Public Health (CDSP).[20] It also appears in the Final Draft on Artificial Conception to be presented to the Council of Ministers in December 1987. The reason given by the council is that semen is *res extra commercium*, in other words semen, like body parts and some other things, is incapable in law of being bought and sold as an item of commerce. That view, which I support, would therefore rule out payments being made to the donors; but it would not prevent the refunding of travelling expenses.

However, semen *donation*, strictly so called, is not by any means a universal practice – probably most donors are paid. The BMA Panal recommended remuneration,[21] and payment is a feature of the AID service in the USA.[22] Donors are paid in Australia and Canada[23] and also in some European countries, for example Spain and Denmark.[24] Where the practice is to pay donors the term 'donor' is a misnomer, and one writer has suggested that they be called 'sperm vendors',[25] but because the term 'donor' is so firmly established it will probably continue to be used.

Two points can be made about the use of the term 'donor' where the 'donor' is paid. The term 'donor' suggests that the giver is doing something for the benefit of humanity, on the analogy of the blood donor. It might therefore be suggested that he should be given some special protection, which would not be appropriate where the transaction is entered into only for the money. The non-legal problems of paid blood 'donors' have been highlighted by Richard Titmus in his book *The Gift Relationship*.[26] The other point is that if the 'donor' is paid it would be wrong to regard him as a patient and obtain his signature on a 'consent' form. He is not consenting to anything but is contracting with the doctor.[27] This may seem a fine legal distinction but it has some bearing on the liability of the 'donor' if the relationship between him and the doctor is that of buyer and seller in a contract of sale. If semen is sold, the contract would be governed by any legislation dealing with defective or dangerous products, which might permit the doctor to sue the donor if the semen was unsuitable. The relation-ship of a paid 'donor' to the doctor might seem to be wholly different from that between the seller and purchaser of, say, a pair of shoes, but unless there is some reason in principle why semen cannot be sold, then the relationships in both instances are governed by rules on contracts of sale, and those governing defec-tive products. This matter has never been decided, but there has been litigation on the related topic of blood donation. It has been said that the supply of blood by a blood bank to a hospital is a sale, because the transaction is purely commercial and involves only the one commodity.[28] By contrast, even where a patient in a hospital has paid for blood which was supplied, the contract between the hospital and the patient is nevertheless not a sale,[29] because what is supplied to a patient is not the blood, bandages and so on but other treatment, for example a surgical operation, of which these other things are incidental, albeit necessary. Applying these anal-ogies to semen donation one might conclude that the transaction between the doctor and the patient is not a sale because what the patient contracts for is a service – artificial insemination. On the other hand the arrangement between the donor and the doctor could be a sale, since there are no other services provided.

If it is established that the transaction between the donor and the doctor is a sale, it would be important to decide what are the obligations of the parties. It is highly unlikely that these will have been expressly set out by either party; therefore there might be some debate about what each party is undertaking. However most people would anticipate that the donor would give certain under-takings or assurances about his physical and genetic health, which would include an honest account of his family history. In addition he would be expected to agree to surrender all rights to any child born to the recipient. (There would be considerable doubt about the enforceability of such a condition.) The doctor would undertake to pay the donor and not to reveal his identity. He might also agree to inform the donor of any defect which tests revealed. The consequence of classifying the agreement between the donor and the doctor as a sale would be that the doctor could sue the donor and vice versa if either party failed to implement its conditions. A simple example would be where the doctor failed to make payment. More contentious would be a claim by the doctor that the semen was 'sub-standard' or 'defective'.

Under Scots and Roman-Dutch law it would be possible for a third party, for example the child, to sue the donor if his failure to perform the contract resulted in loss, injury or damage to the child.[30] In many legal systems, for example England and the Anglo-American jurisdictions, there is the doctrine of privity of contract, which means that, as a general rule, only the parties to the contract can sue on it. Hence it would not be possible for the child to sue the doctor in respect of a breach of his contractual obligations.[31]

The fact that the child might not be able to sue the donor in contract would not prevent his suing the donor in respect of injuries which he suffered. He could base his action in delict/tort, because that right of action is independent of any rights under a contract. This point is dealt with more fully below, under 'Legal implications'.

Selection

Selecting suitable persons from among those recruited is a two-part process. The first is to identify the qualities which donors must possess; and the second is to screen all donors to exclude those who do not have those qualities.

Qualities Those who have written on this subject have listed a number of desirable features, but most give as their principal requirements that the donor (a) be physically fit; and (b) have semen of good quality.[32] Although it is possible to draw up a long list of 'qualities',[33] an important consideration, especially where fresh semen is used, is the donor's availability, and that may determine whether the donor is a medical student or not. Thus it is probably true to say that where the AID service is provided at a teaching hospital the majority of donors will be medical students, but where the service is not so linked the donors will probably be married and come from a variety of backgrounds.

Examination of the donor The next step is to exclude donors who would not be regarded as suitable. The importance of this cannot be underestimated. The object of this screening is to exclude those who might transmit something harmful, either to the recipient or, more probably, to the child. It will also exclude those who are just not healthy. Nor surprisingly concern has been expressed about the possibility of a donor who suffers from acquired immune deficiency syndrome (AIDS) transmitting this to the child.[34] After four Australian women were reported to have been infected the Department of Health and Social Security in the UK introduced a screening programme in 1985.[35]

The first point to consider is whether a full medical examination is desirable or necessary. Opinions vary, but at the Fourth Study Group of the RCOG one contributor was clearly of the view that there was little to be gained from such an examination.[36] He said, 'The number of significant inheritable disorders that hide beneath clothes and are detectable by physical examination must be very few.' His practice is to take a full personal and family history and he suggested that the good faith of the potential donors is a much surer guarantee of what he termed 'genetic cleanliness'. He also pointed out that a 'history of producing healthy children with one woman in no way rules out the possibility of fathering an abnormal child with another woman'.[37]

If the prospective donor is honest, medical histories would permit the doctor to exclude persons with a family history of any condition which is genetically-determined, or a recurrent family history of illness or birth defects. It would also rule out someone with a history of mental illness.

In Australia, 'the extent to which a donor is clinically examined varies widely from clinic to clinic'.[38] The Australian experience also demonstrates the need for trust. Family and personal medical histories are taken, but it is not possible to check all the information that is given. However according to one writer, 'It is thought unlikely that anyone who is sufficiently motivated to volunteer to be a donor would give false information for the small financial gain.'[39]

This family history is particularly important for the genetic screening of donors. The donor must therefore give honest answers. However, as the authors of a US survey suggest, 'the financial incentive to a donor may make this procedure less reliable'. The analogy which they use is again that of the paid blood donor.[40] In France under the CECOS system, potential donors are carefully studied, and this includes taking a personal and family history and submitting them to a physical examination.[41]

Apart from giving these histories, and possibly undergoing a medical examination, the donor's blood will be grouped, and he will be given tests for venereal disease. The object of the blood grouping is to prevent Rhesus incompatibility, but the result will be that the blood groups of many children will differ from those of the husband or male partner of their mother.[42]

The tests for venereal disease can conveniently be made at the initial contact with the donor, but it has to be borne in mind that they may take some time to conclude, and do not preclude the possibility of future infection. In order to ensure against that, it might seem appropriate to require the donor to be tested on each occasion. This has been suggested by one writer in respect of gonorrhoea[43] but the problem is that this may offend the donor and so make him less willing to participate. One way round this would be to use only frozen semen and to examine every specimen before use;[44] but not every centre has access to a semen bank.

Examination of semen   Central to the selection of suitable donors is an examination of the semen to ensure that it is of suitable quality. Most doctors require their donors to be 'highly fertile' but this means different things to different doctors. In Australia, while every clinic has its own standards, 'overall they are similar. A sperm count of at least 80×10^6/ml and a motility of at least 60 per cent with good forward progression, are the basic criteria.'[45] In other words a sufficient quantity of lively sperm is necessary. In France a sperm count of at least 50×10^6/ml is required and a motility of at least 40 per cent after freezing.[46] Other figures range from 40×10^6/ml to 70×10^6/ml.[47]

Screening for genetic disease[48]   The subject of genetic disease is some-what complex and what follows is a very simplified account. It is necessary to make some mention of the topic; otherwise terms like 'genetic screening' make little or no sense. Potential AID couples will wish to ensure, as far as possible, that the donor does not transmit anything in his genetic make-up which might harm the child or the child's offspring.

Genetic disease can be broadly classified in three groups. The first are caused by 'chromosomal diseases' – having an irregular number of chromosomes or by changes in particular chromosomes. Chromosomes are the genetic material which make up the cells of the human body and a normal cell has twenty-three pairs of chromosomes. In the next category are diseases caused by an abnormality in one of the genes which make up the chromosomes. These are called 'single gene' diseases. And in the third category are diseases which result from more than one gene being affected; these are known as 'polygenic' diseases.

Chromosomal diseases   Some of these are caused when the number of chromosomes is more or less than the normal forty-six (the twenty-three pairs). A well-known example is Down's Syndrome (mongolism) where the affected person usually has forty-seven chromosomes (trisomy); but some cases of mongolism are caused by part of one chromosome breaking off and attaching itself to another (translocation). While is it known that the older the parents are at the time of conception the more likely they are to have a Down's child, it is not possible at present to carry out tests prior to conception, though a test can be done during pregnancy. Where AID is being contemplated the best that can be done is to ensure that donors are younger rather than older.

'Single gene' diseases Two of the chromosomes are sex chromosomes and some genetic diseases are caused by abnormal genes on one of the chromosomes. Two such diseases are Hunter Syndrome and Lesch-Nyham Syndrome, both of which cause mental retardation. At present it is not possible to screen persons in order to determine whether their children are likely to be adversely affected. The most that can be done is to carry out tests during pregnancy to detect any abnormality in the foetus.

Other 'single gene' genetic diseases are not linked with the sex chromosomes. They can be divided into two classes – dominant and recessive. In a disease which is caused by a dominant gene, each person who suffers from it has a 50 per cent chance of passing it on to his children. One such disease is Huntington's Chorea which causes a progressive destruction of the brain and premature death. At present techniques are being developed to allow some of these diseases to be detected during pregnancy.

Most of the diseases caused by single genes are recessive diseases. Usually these cannot be detected prior to conception, but there are exceptions, for example Tay-Sachs disease which causes blindness. Greater success has been achieved in detecting these diseases in early pregnancy.

Polygenic diseases These are caused by a combination of defective genes and since there is no one determining factor it is not possible to screen for them prior to conception. Many however can be detected during pregnancy.

In the last year or so a new process has been developed for the early detection of hereditary disorders. This is chorionic biopsy and its aim is to detect foetuses which may suffer from Huntington's Chorea, thalassaemia, phenylketonuria and Down's Syndrome. This procedure has the advantage that the defect can be identified in the foetus at ten weeks, rather than between sixteen and nineteen weeks as at present.

From this brief outline it is clear – at present – that little can be gained by screening all donors. It would not be of significant benefit to screen all recipients as well as donors, and both programmes would be expensive. One must balance the potential benefit of a screening programme against the cost of mounting it. If that is done it would not seem profitable to have one, but as more tests are discovered it may become profitable, and perhaps even necessary, to have such a programme.

In a survey carried out by Curie-Cohen *et al.* among practitioners in the USA, 711 physicians likely to perform AI were asked to participate. Of the 471 responses 379 actually provided AI. However some disturbing facts emerged. The authors concluded that 'most screening was performed by physicians who were not trained for the task'.[49] They gave a number of examples. Doctors had been asked to produce a list of traits which would result in a donor being rejected. However the conditions which the doctors listed had a variety of causes. They included Tay-Sachs disease which is a recessive condition but for which there is a test to identify carriers. Another recessive condition was mentioned, cystic fibrosis; for that there was no test. The list also included Huntington's Chorea, which is a dominant characteristic, and mental retardation which is polygenic. It is not possible to test donors to find out if they are carriers of these conditions.

Over 70 per cent of physicians said that they would reject a donor who had a haemophiliac in his family. This condition is sex-linked with the X chromosome and it could not be passed on unless the donor himself was a sufferer. Other points of criticism were that while 92 per cent would reject a donor with Down's Syndrome, only 12.5 per cent examined the donor's karyotype to determine whether the condition existed. (It must be observed here that views differ on the benefits of karyotyping.)[50] The most alarming revelation was that 94 per cent would reject a carrier of Tay-sachs disease but less than 1 per cent tested for the condition. Only 29 per cent of physicians carried out any biochemical tests other than blood-typing and the tests which were done were primarily in respect of communicable diseases.

The authors concluded that 'while prevention of genetic disease is a goal, it cannot be accomplished by the means currently in use. The findings also raise serious questions about the ability of these physicians to act as genetic counsellors.' While the report did not cover all those practising AID in the USA, and it would be improper to suggest that the same disturbing revelations would be made if a similar survey was done elsewhere, nevertheless some of the points made are sufficiently important to prompt those who provide an AID service to consider whether their standards are as high as they could be. Some of the activities disclosed in the report could, for example, result in the doctor being liable for professional negligence.

However despite the bleak, and in some respects alarming, picture painted by Curie-Cohen, in a survey of the world-wide incidence of congenital abnormalities in AID services for the twenty-five years to 1973 the figure was less than 1 per cent in the 3000 reported births, which is lower than average.[51]

Guidelines

Some have thought it necessary or desirable to have some guidelines, in order to avoid the pitfalls disclosed by Curie-Cohen or to ensure high standards.

With the exception of the State of Oregon and the Yugoslavian Republics of Slovenia and Croatia, there is no legislation dealing with the selection of donors. The Oregon statute prohibits semen donation if the donor 'has any disease or defect known by him to be transmissible by genes; or knows or has any reason to know he has a venereal disease'.[52] The law in the Republic of Slovenia provides that 'the donor shall be mentally and physically healthy', and the doctor is under an obligation not to use the semen from a donor who would not be able to marry the woman because of their consanguinity.[53] The Republic of Croatia does not mention consanguinity, but otherwise the provision is similar, namely 'the donor of semen may only be a healthy man'.[54]

In New York, Israel and Switzerland there are guidelines laid down by the health authorities, but these do not have the force of law. The New York City Health Code provision is as follows:'A person who is afflicted with a venereal disease, tuberculosis, brucellosis or who has any congenital disease or defect shall not be used as a donor of seminal fluid for artificial insemination.'[55] The rules of the Ministry of Health of Israel are more detailed:

Sperm from a donor will not be taken, not be received and not be used for the purpose of artificial insemination in any of the following cases:

(i) the sperm is not healthy;
(ii) prior to the donation, the donor did not have a general medical examination, including physical examination, chest X-ray and blood-test;
(iii) the donor suffers from venereal disease, from tuberculosis, from infection of the sexual organ or of the sperm, or from a disease which may affect the woman or the child;
(iv) the donor is married.[56]

The following guidelines have been laid down by the Swiss Academy of Medical Sciences:

(i)   the physician must be guided by 'medical considerations', 'but should also, as far as possible, make sure that the well being of the future child is guaranteed in a comprehensive manner';

(ii) the sperm donor must give his consent for its use. Written consent must also be obtained from the woman and her husband or 'in the case of a lasting partnership, her partner';

(iii) the physician must make 'appropriate inquiries and examinations of the donor to avoid transmission of a hereditary disease or other risks to the woman and the future child'. If necessary, the physician can obtain cooperation from the human genetic institutes. 'The semen of the same donor should not be used again in the same place (to avoid kinship of blood etc.)';

(iv) the physician should 'choose a donor whose child could be considered a child born to the couple who want the child';

(v)   the identity of the woman and the donor must be kept secret;

(vi) semen shall be donated without payment, but expenses, such as travelling expenses, can be refunded.[57]

Matching

At the initial meeting with the potential donor a record will probably be made of his race, height, eye colour, hair colour and general build. It is possible to ensure that these characteristics of the donor are broadly compatible with those of the husband. However, while most doctors will probably make some attempt to match these features, it is not necessary to be particularly concerned about the matter, simply because children of the same biological parents vary so much. One practitioner has said that, at first, he always tried to match the physical characteristics of the donor with those of the husband, but later his experience showed that 'patients are not fastidious about the matching and prefer to become pregnant as soon as possible'.[58]

While it may be correct to say this about physical features, other factors may be of some concern to the recipients. Clearly race is important, but a doctor is unlikely to use a donor from a different race. Couples may wish the donor to be intelligent and some may wish him to be of the same religious persuasion as themselves. On the question of intelligence, most doctors do not make any formal effort to match intelligence but they would try to avoid gross discrepancies.[59] There may be a problem where the potential parents are of below average intelligence. One distinguished geneticist has said that there would be no advantage in providing a 'dim child for the satisfaction of dim parents',[60] and in any event there are numerous instances of 'dim' parents with bright children.

As far as religion is concerned, there seems little point in securing a donor of the same religious persuasion as the couple, unless they specifically requested this. An exception would probably be made in the case of Jewish couples where it is desirable that the donor is also Jewish; but this is matching, not on the grounds of religion but on race and the associated physical characteristics.

Legal implications

Of these activities – recruitment, selection and matching – the last two are probably of greater legal significance than the first, because they result in the choice of a particular donor for the couple. If an unsuitable donor is not excluded, that may cause loss or damage to the child and/or the couple and result in an action being raised against the doctor. The child might raise an action on the ground that it has been born with some physical or mental handicap which, it argues, can be traced to the donor. The couple might raise an action against the doctor if, for example, he selected a black donor for them when they were white. A claim of this nature is within the ambit of the law of delict or tort.

The most likely cause of action would be the alleged failure by the doctor to exclude an unsuitable donor, namely that he had been negligent. This is a very important topic on which there is an immense literature in the UK and USA alone, and no two systems of law will be alike in all respects. Accordingly we give a brief statement of the law only as it exists in the UK and USA. (In the USA it would be possible to raise an action for breach of contract, but in the UK there is no contractual relationship between the doctor and an NHS patient.[61] There would be a contract however where the AID was not provided under the NHS.)

In the UK and the USA, the principles are broadly the same. The law requires a person to take reasonable care to avoid acts or omissions which he can reasonably foresee will be likely to cause injury to someone else.[62] A simple example would be a driver who injures a passenger or pedestrian. The law requires everyone to drive with reasonable care. If a person does not drive with this degree of care and as a result causes someone injury, he will be liable if a court takes the view that he should have foreseen the injury.

If an issue arises as to whether a person has been negligent or not, his conduct is usually judged by that of the hypothetical 'reasonable man'. This person has been variously described as 'the man on the Clapham omnibus' and 'the man who takes the magazines at home and in the evening pushes the lawnmower in his shirt sleeves'.[63]

There is considerable debate about the advantage of such descriptions, but it is clear that this standard of the reasonable man is not appropriate when what is to be judged is the conduct of someone with special knowledge or skill, such as a doctor.[64] It could not be argued that because the man on the Clapham omnibus would make a botch of a surgical operation a surgeon would escape liability if he did the same thing. What is required of professionals is that they demonstrate the skill which is usually possessed by members of their profession who are in good standing.[65] Accordingly if it is suggested that a doctor has been negligent he will be judged by the standards of his profession.

However it does not follow that because something has gone wrong the doctor has been negligent. Mistakes do happen, even when people are being as careful as is humanly possible. Furthermore a doctor will not necessarily be negligent simply because he has not acted in accordance with the view or practice of a majority of his profession. There are, and must be room for, different schools of thought, and if a doctor follows one school rather than another he will be judged in accordance with the thinking of that school. That school of thought must of course be that of at least a respectable minority of the profession.

Turning now to the specific elements of a claim based on negligence, the plaintiff (pursuer) must prove four things:

(a)   that there existed a duty of care owed by the defendant (defender)to the plaintiff;
(b)   that the defendant was in breach of that duty of care;
(c)   that the breach caused loss, injury or damage;
(d)   that that loss, injury or damage was foreseeable.[66]

When an action is raised on the basis of a doctor's involvement in AID, each of these four elements would have to be established by the claimant; in other words it is not for the doctor to show that his conduct was free from blame. In the UK and USA there would be little doubt that the doctor who performs AID owes a duty of care not to do anything or omit to do something, the effect of which might be to cause harm to the child. However the other elements of the claim are more difficult.

Having established that there was a duty of care, the next thing would be to establish that the doctor was in breach of that duty. To succeed it would have to be shown that in the processes of screening or matching (and more probably the former) the doctor did something or, more likely, omitted to do something which a reasonably proficient doctor would have done, or would not have omitted to do. Alternatively if it could be shown that although the doctor complied with the requirements of his profession the omission was nevertheless such an obvious one as to make the doctor culpable, then liability may follow. These points are best illustrated by two examples – a failure of the doctor to test the donor for syphilis and a failure to test for Tay-Sachs disease.

If the child's claim is that he suffered injury because the donor suffered from syphilis but this was not detected because he was not tested by the doctor, the child would be able to adduce evidence from other doctors to the effect that it is standard practice to do such a test. Accordingly if a doctor failed to carry out such a test he would have failed to comply with the standards of the profession, and hence would be in breach of the duty of care.

The example of Tay-Sachs disease is slightly different. It might be shown that the doctor failed to carry out such a test, but, as the Curie-Cohen survey demonstrates, less than 1 per cent of the doctors covered by the survey actually performed the test.[67] Thus even although the doctor did not perform a test he would be following the practice of reasonably proficient members of the profession. However it would still be open to show that the failure to test was an obvious omission. One Scottish judge said that, if a claimant was adopting this argument, he would have to show 'that the course the doctor adopted is one which no professional man of ordinary skill would have taken if he had been acting with ordinary care'.[68] The claimant might therefore succeed if he could show that a failure to test for Tay-Sachs disease came into this category. There are no reported decisions on this point, but the survey carried out by Curie-Cohen would be a telling factor. Of the physicians questioned 95 per cent would reject a carrier of the disease, and so it would seem appropriate to test the donor for this condition. If therefore the doctor failed to carry out the test, this could be said to be a course which no doctor exercising ordinary care would adopt.

An analogy can be seen in the case of *Ravenis v. Detroit General Hospital*[69] which involved a corneal transplant. The cornea were infected and Ravenis was rendered totally and permanently blind. He sued the hospital and the doctor who had removed the donor's eyes. The jury found in favour of the doctor, but against the hospital. They had heard evidence to the effect that if the deceased had suffered from certain types of illnesses his cornea would generally be regarded as unsuitable for transplantation. The court stated that whoever had to make the decision about the suitability of the cornea would have to know the donor's medical history. The hospital was negligent in that it had failed to set up any procedure which would have made the records available to the doctor. The hospital's omission could be regarded as something so obvious that nobody exercising reasonable care would have acted in the way in which it did.

Having demonstrated the existence of a duty of care and a breach of this duty, two further things have to be shown. The first is that the breach caused injury and the second that the breach was of a foreseeable kind. Although the issues of causation and forseeability are difficult and have exercised the minds of lawyers for some time,[70] they are considered here together. They can be illustrated by again taking the example of syphilis. The child's claim might be that he was born blind as the result of a syphilitic infection. In order to succeed in such an action he would have to show that the blindness was caused by the syphilis and not, for example, by a hereditary factor. Having done that, it would be necessary to show that the blindness was a foreseeable consequence of the infection, in other words that the doctor should have anticipated that if a donor suffered from syphilis this might cause blindness in the child. It is not enough to prove that there was cause and effect. It must also be shown that this should have been foreseen. The causal link might have been revealed only at some later stage.

The Congenital Disabilities (Civil Liability) Act 1976 applies where a child is born disabled as a result of an occurrence which either affected the ability of one of its parents to have a normal healthy child, or affected the mother during the pregnancy or the child in the course of its birth.[71] It is perhaps questionable whether the Act would apply to a disorder which resulted from a failure to screen the donor properly. The Act follows a Report of the (English) Law Commission;[72] but when the Scottish Law Commission considered the issue[73] it was felt that legislation was unnecessary in Scotland, since ante-natal injuries could be the subject of an action at common law. There is nothing at common law which would indicate that a failure to screen a donor which resulted in damage to the child could not be the subject of such an action in Scotland.

Success in any action would not be easily achieved. For that reason, among others, there has been considerable debate for a number of years about the need to replace the 'fault' system just described.[74] It is not appropriate to pursue this much further here. It is enough to say that there are alternatives, the most radical of which is a state benefits scheme for physical and mental disability. Such a system operates in New Zealand and benefits are paid to those who suffer whatever the cause of the suffering provided that it results from 'accident' and irrespective of fault.[75]

If the action was based on contract rather than delict, it might be difficult in some jurisdictions for the child to sue because he was clearly not a party to the contract. If however the child could sue on contract or his 'parents' did, the result would be the same as in an action based on delict/tort. The doctor would be in breach of contract if he did not screen the donor properly and his failure resulted in damage to the child. The child could sue in respect of his damage and the parents could sue for their loss also.

Conclusion

There are features of the recruiting, selecting and matching of donors which ought to be examined carefully in the light of the Curie-Cohen report. Nevertheless the reported incidence of mental and physical handicap in AID children is low, and even where it has occurred it does not follow that this is attributable to fault on the part of the doctors.

What is of prime importance is that all who are involved in providing AID attain the highest possible standards. These could be laid down by statute but are perhaps best left to the medical profession within particular countries. Other groups may be involved in recruitment, selection and matching, but it is the donor's medical condition which is more likely to be at issue in any claim for damages. It is therefore for the doctor to ensure that the donor is not unsuitable for the task. Failure to do so could expose the doctor to court action.

11 Selection and counselling of recipients

The selection and counselling of recipients, like that of donors, demands considerable skill. Although the process raises many ethical and sociological issues there are fewer legal implications than in the selection of donors. Again the principles governing recipients of AID apply equally to egg and embryo donation.

In this chapter, unless the context indicates otherwise, the assumption is that it is a married couple who are requesting AID. The provision of AID for unmarried couples, single persons, lesbians or even transsexuals, does not for the most part raise any special legal problems. Nevertheless these matters have been discussed and something is said about them later.

Before selecting a couple for AID their doctor will probably have assumed or decided (a) that the man is incapable of fathering a child, or it is undesirable that he should do so; and (b) that there is no bar to conception in the woman. At some stage decisions will also be made about whether the couple are sufficiently informed about AID, whether they are reconciled to it and whether they are likely to prove suitable parents.

The first legal issue is whether there is any liability if the doctor's assumptions or decisions about the man or woman are wrong. For example, if it turns out that the man is capable of fathering a child or that the woman is not able to conceive, would the fact that the doctor recommended AID give rise to liability because the couple had been advised they were unlikely to have a child naturally?

A second issue is whether the couple would have any redress against the doctor if the child is born with a physical or mental handicap. This is dealt with in Chapter 10 and nothing further need be added here. The third point is whether a doctor might be liable in law if he gives inaccurate or incomplete advice to the couple about AID. This involves a discussion of consent.

Before discussing these points, it is useful to sketch in the medical background in the hope that this will indicate how the legal issues might arise. We shall look first at the decision that a man is incapable of fathering a child, then at the advice that he should not father a child and finally at the decision about the wife's ability to conceive.

Inability to father a child

The conclusion that someone is incapable of fathering a child should have been reached only after detailed examination, including, usually, several seminal analyses.[1] These may reveal that the man is not producing any sperm, or no live sperm. In such a case a doctor can be quite unequivocable that the man will not be able to father a child.

Where the man's semen contains some live sperm but his sperm count is below average (oligospermia) however, the doctor has to decide whether it is probable or improbable that the man will father a child; but he cannot be certain. One of the difficulties is that views differ on how low a sperm count must be before a man can be described as oligospermic.[2] Given these differences of opinion, a couple might consult one doctor and decide to undergo AID because in his opinion the husband is oligospermic; whereas another doctor might decline to offer AID to the same couple because in his view the man is not oligospermic, and hence he might father a child. What is more likely is that the doctor would base his assessment on the man's sperm count and the length of time the couple had been trying to have a child, rather than a somewhat arbitrary 'definition' of oligospermia.

Nevertheless, doctors will still have different views on whether a particular man could father a child. The doctor's advice in such circumstances would be an important factor in a couple's decision to undergo AID, rather than try to have a child of their own. Accordingly the issue arises whether a doctor could incur any liability for suggesting AID, when another doctor might not regard the couple as suitable because he did not regard the man as infertile.

It is possible that a couple who had a child by AID might subsequently discover that the husband could father a child. They might therefore raise a court action against the doctor, claiming that the advice he had given about the husband's chances of fathering a child was wrong, that they had followed his advice, and so had been prevented from having the husband's child.

There is no doubt that in the USA there is a limited constitutional right to have a child.[3] There is also a clause to the same effect in the European Convention on Human Rights[4] and there is no UK legislation which would prevent persons having children if they wished. However, these legislative provisions are aimed at prohibitions or restrictions which make it difficult for certain types of persons to have children, for example criminals,[5] or which fetter the discretion of others about whether or not to have children.[6] Accordingly they would not be of assistance to a couple who had had a child by AID and were arguing that AID was unnecessary.

If a couple raised an action against a doctor, in many jurisdictions they would have to base it on negligence. Before the doctor could be made liable, it would have to be proved that he did not act in accordance with the standards of his profession[7] or that what he did was so obviously wrong that, whether or not his professional colleagues also did it, it ought not to have been done.[8]

Although a doctor can be liable for giving negligent advice,[9] an action in respect of allegedly negligent advice about AID is extremely unlikely to succeed. In the first place the advice would probably make it clear that it was not impossible for the man to father a child, but that the possibility was remote. Secondly, and just as important, the couple would be aware of their own unsuccessful attempts to have a family and would have consulted a doctor only because it occurred to them that something was wrong. Even if they could establish that they had relied to a very substantial degree on the medical advice, the doctor would be able to point to colleagues who would have made the same decision and given the same advice as he did.

Advice that it is undesirable that a person should father a child

In this case there is of course nothing to suggest that the husband is incapable of fathering a child. What is being stressed is that there is a risk that if he does father a child he may transmit some disorder to it.

In such a situation the doctor's advice would be that there is a chance that a child or its offspring might suffer from the disorder. For example, if a man suffers from Huntington's Chorea, there is a 50 per cent chance, or 1 in 2, that his children will be affected.[10] The doctor's advice to such a person might be strongly against his fathering a child and AID might therefore be recommended. Should the couple follow that advice they would deprive themselves of having children of their own.

The advice might be questioned at a later stage for a variety of reasons. For example, the couple might ignore the advice and have a child which did not suffer from the particular disorder. (Huntington's Chorea does not manifest itself until later life, but there are other disorders which reveal themselves in early childhood.) Another possibility is that they know of another man who suffers from the same disorder but whose children are not affected. The couple might reconsider the advice and even raise court proceedings against the doctor for failing to give proper advice.

In the USA there has been litigation over alleged failures by doctors to give adequate advice to pregnant women about the effects of a disease or genetic disorder on the foetus.[11] In these cases the doctor had either not given any advice or given advice which, it was argued, was wrong. The women had given birth to children with physical or mental handicaps, and they argued that they ought to have been told about the possibility of handicaps and given the opportunity of an abortion. But these examples are distinguishable from AID, in that the advice in genetic counselling cases may not have been sought before the pregnancy, but would have been asked for or, arguably, should have been given at an early stage in pregnancy. The result of giving proper advice would probably have been a termination of the pregnancy. However, these cases do establish that doctors can be made liable for failing to give advice or for giving inaccurate advice on genetics. Actions of this kind have not yet been raised in the UK, but there is no reason in principle why they should not be successful.[12]

If a man who had been advised not to father children raised an action against the doctor in respect of that advice, his argument would be similar to that put forward by the couple who had been advised about AID where the husband was infertile. It would be slightly different however, in that the man would probably put greater store on the advice of the doctors because he would not necessarily be able to assess the consequences for himself. That would make his prospects of success greater, but he would still have to show that the doctor had been negligent. It is extremely unlikely that he would succeed, because some other doctors would have given the same advice about the risk of inheriting the disorder.

If, therefore, a couple who had been advised to undergo AID because of the husband's infertility, or because he might pass on an inheritable disorder to his children, wished to prove that the advice was wrong and that the doctor had been negligent, they would find this extremely difficult. In this context it should not be forgotten that women who are given AID are usually grateful, especially if they become pregnant. Accordingly they are probably unlikely to challenge advice about the prospects of the husband fathering a child or advice about the risks of doing so.

The ability of the wife to conceive

Having discussed possible liability arising from the advice given to the husband, we turn to the wife. It is obvious that AID would not be successful unless the woman is able to conceive. The wife's ability to conceive is central also to egg and embryo donation. Thus if the husband undergoes tests and examinations to ascertain whether or not he is fertile, or whether it is desirable that he should father a child, it seems appropriate that the wife should do the same. If a wife was not examined she might undergo artificial insemination for some considerable time before she was made aware that she was unable to conceive. She might, with justification, feel aggrieved at the cost and inconvenience which resulted. That of itself suggests it is desirable that the wife undergoes as complete an assessment as her husband.

However, practice varies.[13] Some doctors will provide AID for a woman whose husband is infertile without giving her a detailed examination, unless the woman has had another partner and failed to conceive by him.[14] If having undergone AID for, say, six months the woman does not conceive, these practitioners would then advise that her tubes be X-rayed (HSG); and if she has not conceived after a year, they would recommend laparoscopy, which is a surgical examination of the abdominal cavity including the ovaries, Fallopian tubes and the uterus. The principal reason given for this approach is that neither HSG nor laparoscopy is entirely free from complications.

Another school of thought favours a full initial examination of the woman, possibly including laparoscopy.[15] One writer justifies this on the following grounds:

(1) AID women are older than normal fertile women and may have more hidden pathology;
(2) AID women may be relatively infertile themselves particularly if their husbands, although oligospermic, have reasonable sperm counts;
(3) laparoscopy is relatively free of morbidity in experienced hands;
(4) unsuspected pathology associated with decreased success rates can be accurately identified;
(5) couples undertaking the programme can know their success rates and will accept failure with less frustration;
(6) precious semen is not wasted;
(7) waiting lists are reduced;
(8) costs are reduced where unnecessary visits are eliminated.[16]

These two schools of thought cannot be reconciled but each has its advantages and disadvantages. The first has the merit that the woman can commence AID as soon as possible after infertility or an inheritable trait in her husband is diagnosed, and she is not exposed to even the slightest risk before undergoing AID. The disadvantages are that she may spend some time having AID and might subsequently be advised that she is not able to conceive unless she has some further treatment. She may therefore have incurred considerable expense and wasted donor semen which is never plentiful. The advantages of the alternative approach are clearly spelt out above and need not be repeated. The principal disadvantage is that the woman is exposed to whatever risks attend HSG and laparoscopy.

If a woman suffered injury as the result of laparoscopy she might raise an action against the doctor, which could result in a discussion of the relative merits of the two approaches. This would certainly happen if it was contended that laparoscopy was unnecessary, or that the risks involved far outweighed any inconvenience or loss that the woman might suffer by being artificially inseminated, despite her inability to conceive. The differing practices might also come under scrutiny if an action was raised by a woman who had been given AID without it first being ascertained whether or not she could conceive. Her action might be for recovery of any fees paid for the inseminations and compensation for the time wasted. The balance of opinion seems to favour the more detailed examination of the woman prior to commencing artificial insemination. That however is not conclusive of the matter. It would still be for a court to decide whether one course of action is to be preferred or whether both are acceptable from a legal point of view. If court proceedings were raised and the differing approaches were in issue, it is highly unlikely that a court would take the view that either course is negligent.[17]

Summary

As pointed out earlier, a couple who have been given AID are unlikely to complain about the length of the treatment, especially if it is successful. If a woman did feel so aggrieved that she raised court proceedings, she would probably not succeed, given that one approach to treatment is not necessarily preferable to the other. Undoubtedly a more accurate assessment can be had if the woman undergoes HSG and laparoscopy. These involve some risks, but the risks with laparoscopy seem to be fewer with more experienced doctors.[18] It may therefore be that the way to determine which of the two courses is to be preferred, if either, is to have a controlled analysis of all laparoscopies, whatever their purpose.

The issue of liability on the part of the doctor where the child has a mental or physical handicap has already been discussed. We therefore turn our attention to the question whether a patient is sufficiently informed about AID and is reconciled to it, and the circumstances in which a doctor may be liable for the advice which he gives or fails to give about AID.

Consent

In the course of the discussions between the doctor and the couple there are many things he will want to ask or to find out about them. Equally there are questions they will wish to put to him.

The law requires a patient to give consent to any medical procedure, and AID is no different in this respect from a surgical operation. Before a patient undergoes surgery he must be aware of the reasons why it is necessary and what is entailed, for example the risks which might attend the operation, and the chances of success. A patient who is contemplating AID will want to know whether there are any risks and what chance she has of becoming pregnant. Her consent to undergo AID would not be effective in law unless she was aware of what she was doing and was willing to be artificially inseminated with donor semen. If the consent which is given is not legally effective the giving of AID could amount to an assault, and a claim for negligence might also arise.

Legal requirements for consent

A great deal has been written on this subject[19] and so what is presented here is not the full picture, but it is hoped that the essentials are covered.

There are three requirements for consent to be effective in law:

(a) the consent must be given by someone who is legally competent;
(b) the patient must be given reasonable information about the proposed action;
(c) the consent must be clear, unequivocal and comprehensive.[20]

Before looking at these in more detail, it is useful to say a word about whether consent needs to be in writing.

Need for written consent In law, consent which is given orally or even by a nod of the head is just as effective as written consent. However there are considerable advantages in having written consent. It helps to ensure that the doctor covers all the aspects of AID with each patient and, more important, provides a record, principally for the doctor, of what the patient was told. Should there be any dispute at a later stage about what was or was not said, written consent would be very useful. If that is not available the matter has to be trusted to the memory of the parties, who may not recollect even after a month exactly what was said: the chances of remembering after a year or more are even slimmer.

It might be thought by some that to require written consent indicates that the doctor does not trust the patient. Some patients may react in that way if they are asked to sign a consent form, but the advantages of having written consent far outweigh the disadvantages of possible offence taken by the patient. In any event, as we shall see later, it is preferable to keep the consent form simple and brief, and it might put matters more clearly than the doctor. There may therefore be less reason for a patient to take offence.

We can now return to the requirements for valid consent.

Consent to be given by someone legally capable of giving it

In the UK the law relating to consent to medical procedures on persons under full age[21] or those who are mentally ill[22] is not easily stated. It is highly unlikely that a doctor would provide AID for a person in either category, but if he did the purported consent could be invalid.[23] Since most AID patients are married women, an important question is whether the husband's consent is required before his wife can undergo AID. This has never been decided, but in an English case Lord Justice Denning (as he then was) observed that a sterilization operation required the consent of the other spouse.[24] However that opinion was not essential to the judgment, and it has been questioned.[25] A sterilization is obviously different in character from AID but in practice a doctor would not provide AID for a married woman without her husband's consent.[26]

There seems to be only one statutory provision which expressly requires the consent of the husband to be obtained. Somewhat unexpectedly it is part of the law in the Yugoslavian Republic of Croatia.[27] The Republic of Slovenia also has legislation on AID, but does not have a requirement about consent from the husband.[28] As has been mentioned, there are statutory provisions in Sweden and some of the states in the USA[29] which mention consent, but they deal with the status of children conceived as the result of AID and deem such children to be the legitimate issue of the husband only if he gives his consent to the AID. Strictly therefore, he does not require to give consent to the AID, but if he does not the child will not have the benefit of the statutory presumption. In Israel and Switzerland there is no legislation on the subject, but guidelines have been issued which *inter alia* require doctors to obtain the consent of a woman's husband before carrying out AID.[30] Despite the lack of legislative direction most doctors obtain the written consent of the husband and wife.

The consent form is usually, and ought to be, as simple as possible and should be devoted to the essential points about AID. Some consent forms however purport to deal with other subjects, in particular the status of the child. They contain some or all of the following statements:

(a) that the child conceived by AID is the husband's legitimate child;
(b) that he gives up any right to deny this;
(c) that the child will be his lawful heir for succession purposes.

It is difficult to see why these statements are included in consent forms. Unless the jurisdiction allows a husband to 'acknowledge' or 'recognize' his wife's illegitimate child[31] and the consent form sufficed for this purpose, statements of this type about the child's status will not affect the legal position. If by the law of a particular state an AID child is *illegitimate*, that is not altered simply by the husband stating or agreeing that the child is his *legitimate* child.

The child's status, its rights to maintenance and of succession to the husband's estate on his death, are not matters with which doctors should concern themselves, and for that reason alone statements of this kind are best left out of consent forms.

The patient must be given adequate information

Of all the aspects of consent, this has probably received greatest consideration.[32] In the USA the patient's consent must be 'informed'.[33] This means that there must be a very full disclosure to the patient of all material matters before he makes up his mind. In England at least, this is not the standard and what the patient is told is judged by the standards of the medical profession. So whether a patient has been adequately informed will be judged by what other doctors would have told that particular patient.[34] It is of particular importance to decide what to tell the patient about AID and the implications of the treatment. While information about the diagnosis of infertility may not be of such significance in AID, there are other matters which would have to be dealt with before the patient could be described as having been given reasonable information. The patient would clearly want to know about the prospects of success and whether AID is more risky than natural conception. The doctor should therefore explain how donors are recruited and selected and what attempts, if any, are made to match the husband and the donor. It would also be important to point out that a pregnancy resulting from AID entails no greater risk than any other pregnancy; indeed the risks may be fewer. Some indication should also be given about the chances of a woman becoming pregnant by AID. All these matters are dealt with in the booklet for patients issued by the Royal College of Obstetricians and Gynaecologists, to which a consent form is attached. If the patient has read that booklet, then there is little scope for suggesting that the patient was not given a reasonable amount of information on which to make a decision.

When the issue of consent has come before the courts in the UK, the approach has been to hold that where the proposed medical treatment or procedure has been explained in general terms to the patient who thereafter agrees to it, that amounts to real consent. If there is no consent, the doctor commits an assault on the patient. Whether the consent is 'real' depends on the particular patient, and whether the nature of the treatment, risks and so on have been explained properly is to be judged by the standards of the medical profession. If they have not been so explained the doctor has been negligent.[35] In either case the patient may claim damages. An important distinction is that where the claim is based on assault, the patient may prove this by the evidence of lay witnesses, for example the patient's spouse or other relative who was present at the material time. But where the claim is based on negligence the claimant must bring expert evidence to demonstrate that the doctor departed in some way from the practice of his profession or that there was an obvious omission. The courts have adopted both approaches.[36]

Consent must be clear, unequivocal and comprehensive

There is no reason why a patient's consent to AID should be challenged on the ground that the information provided was unclear, or equivocal or not comprehensive. AID is not difficult to explain, nor should it be difficult to understand. To be comprehensive the consent should cover all the essential features of the treatment, which is not difficult in AID. Some doctors who are aware of the requirement about comprehensiveness include in the consent form a clause which purports to exempt them from liability should something go wrong, for example a child born with some handicap. The advantage of such a clause is that it might dissuade someone from raising an action against the doctor if something untoward did happen. However, there is a disadvantage in that such a clause might give rise to doubts in the mind of the patient about the risks involved and make her more worried than she need be, and it would not prevent an action by the child. If the doctor adheres to the standards of his profession he has little to fear if a court action is raised.

If a patient does give birth to a handicapped child and feels that the doctor has been negligent, there is no guarantee that she will be deterred by the clause in the consent form. She might decide to challenge the consent on any of the grounds mentioned above. It is preferable to keep consent forms as short as possible, and so clauses which purport to deal with liability ought to be omitted.

While it is highly unlikely that a patient would challenge the consent she gave for AID, if such a challenge was made it would most likely be on the grounds that the consent was not informed, either because the doctor omitted to mention something of importance or because he did not explain it properly. The prospects of a successful challenge diminish if written consent has been obtained. Consent is best obtained after the patient has been given a full, but nevertheless simple, explanation in writing of what AID is about, and an opportunity to ask any further questions which may occur to her.

AID for other than married couples

There is little doubt that in the UK, AID is usually provided only for married couples, but in some clinics the service may be extended to cohabiting couples and perhaps also single women and lesbians. In France the national AID service as at 1980 did not provide AID for other than married women.[37] In the USA, while many doctors will provide AID for unmarried women, there is a fear that this may be illegal in some states.[38] The legal issues which arise from the provision of AID to unmarried women are, in the main, the same as where married women are involved. The responsibility in law arising from recruitment and so on of donors is no different, nor is the need to counsel the recipient and obtain her consent to the insemination. Clearly one difference is that any legislation which deals with the status of the AID child would not apply to unmarried women, and their AID children would inevitably be illegitimate.

The issue which frequently arises in this context is whether AID ought to be provided only to married women. This is primarily a social and ethical issue and not a legal one, but there are some legislative provisions which have a bearing on the matter. Both the Universal Declaration of Human Rights[39] and the European Convention on Human Rights[40] provide that everyone has the right to marry and found a family. It could be argued that a single woman, a lesbian or a transsexual has the right under these provisions to have children by AID, but only if the right to marry and the right to found a family can be separated. This point has been discussed in the USA in relation to the constitutionality of refusing to provide AID to unmarried women.[41] The US Supreme Court in *Eisenstadt v. Baird*[42] held that a state law which prohibited the provision of contraceptives to unmarried persons violated the equal protection clause of the 14th Amendment to the Constitution and it has been argued that to refuse AID to unmarried women is also an infringement.[43]

In jurisdictions which have legislation on sex discrimination the provisions may be wide enough to encompass a refusal to provide AID to unmarried women. The Human Rights Commission Act 1979 of New Zealand is wide enough,[44] but in the UK the Sex Discrimination Act 1975 is not, since it deals only with discrimination on the grounds of sex and the only provision dealing with discrimination against married women relates to employment.[45]

In the UK therefore it is not illegal to refuse to supply AID to the unmarried. The arguments for and against such a provision are outside the scope of this book. However, if resources are scarce, there will probably be a tendency to favour married women.

12 Other uses of artificial insemination

Artificial insemination after death

Mention has been made of the possibility of using fresh or frozen semen for artificial insemination. Semen may be preserved as an insurance against future debility or infertility, or for use after a vasectomy, for example where the man remarries. The semen of some American astronauts was preserved because it was feared they might be adversely affected by exposure to radiation.[1] As a general rule no legal issues arise from decision to use frozen rather than fresh semen, but where the semen is used after the death of the person who provided it, this does give rise to complex legal problems.

Human semen can now be preserved for a considerable time – up to ten years has been achieved in the USA – without affecting its potential.[2] It would therefore be possible for a woman to conceive a child long after the death of the person who produced the semen. Such a person might be an anonymous donor, or the woman's cohabiting partner, or her husband. In 1977 it was reported that the cartoonist Kim Casali had given birth to a child sixteen months after its father's death, using semen of his which had been frozen.[3] More recently a Frenchwoman raised court proceedings to enable her to be inseminated with semen from her deceased husband. She succeeded in obtaining the semen but failed to become pregnant.[4] In June 1985 an Englishwoman, Sonia Palmer, applied to St Mary's Hospital, Manchester to be inseminated in this way.[5] The matter was referred to the hospital's ethical committee, but because it is confidential their decision is not known.

Consideration is given first to the use of a donor's semen after his death, then the use of a cohabitee's semen, and finally the use of a husband's semen.

Use of donor's semen after the donor's death

The legal implications of using a donor's semen after his death are, to a large extent, the same as those which arise from its use during his lifetime. The principal legal issues are first whether it would provide a woman's husband with grounds for divorce if the insemination was performed without his consent, and secondly whether the child conceived as the result of AID is regarded in law as the husband's child and whether it would have a right to maintenance from the husband and to succeed to his estate.

There are however three issues peculiar to the use of semen after the donor's death: (a) whether he had agreed to this use; (b) whether his legal representatives could give authority for such use; and (c) whether any children conceived from this semen would be entitled to share in his estate.

The first issue has never arisen and is probably unlikely to arise. If it became known that semen from a donor was being used after his death and someone, for example his wife, objected to this, the matter could be resolved quite simply by referring to any express consent which the donor may have given. He may, for example, have consented to the use of his semen without imposing any time limit. In the absence of such consent, however, authority to use a donor's semen would terminate on his death. If the donor's semen was being used after death without the necessary authority, any of his representatives could object and request that the practice cease. If it did not, then a court would grant an order requiring compliance with the representative's wishes.

The second issue is whether the representatives of a deceased donor can authorize the use of his semen, on the analogy of the use of certain parts of the body for transplant purposes. There are a number of possible objections to this suggestion. A purported authorization might not come within the legislation on the use of human tissue after death, principally because the semen will generally have been obtained from the deceased prior to his death and its use may therefore be regulated by the consent he gave. It is however possible to obtain semen from a deceased person; but if representatives intended to use it, that use would probably not be within the legislative provisions on the use of human tissue after death, since the object of such legislation is to encourage research.[6] This second objection is a formidable one and medical practitioners would probably not wish to be involved in such a practice.

The third issue is whether any children conceived with the donor's semen after his death could claim against his estate. This arises most acutely where it is the semen of a deceased husband which is used; but there would be little doubt that children conceived posthumously by a donor are his illegitimate children, and if the law recognizes claims by illegitimate children, an AID child would have a claim. As was said in the context of the succession rights of AID children, this might raise problems when winding up the donor's estate unless there was legislation which severed all legal links between the donor and the child.

Use of cohabitee's semen after death

This possibility raises exactly the same issues as the use of donor semen, but whereas the identity of the donor would not normally be revealed to the recipient, that would not be so where the woman used her cohabitee's semen. The important point would then be whether any children would have a claim on the man's estate. As the law currently stands they are his illegitimate children and so they might have a claim on his estate.

These two issues also arise and are considered in connection with the use of a husband's semen after death.

Artificial insemination using a husband's semen after his death

This practice raises two main issues – the status of the child and the consequences for the husband's estate of the birth of such a child. There is little doubt that in the USA and the UK a child conceived as a result of AIH while the husband is still alive is legitimate. The legislation in the UK provides that where a decree of nullity of marriage is granted in respect of a voidable marriage any child which would have been the legitimate child of the parties to the marriage had it been dissolved instead of being annulled shall be regarded as their legitimate child.[8] This clearly envisages a child conceived during the marriage, even if born thereafter, but the statute does not apply to a child conceived after the husband's death.

As the husband's death terminates the marriage, any child which could not have been conceived during the subsistence of the marriage is illegitimate. To avoid this conclusion the definition of marriage would have to be altered to take account of the possibility of a child being conceived after death. One writer at least, however, feels that this conclusion is inequitable and asks:

> Would you sitting on any Bench you care to name, put this stigma on the child thus conceived and deprive him of his share in his grand-father's estate, and bring down social obloquy on the courageous widow . . . if you would still rule for illegitimacy can you be sure that the appropriate legislature with all deliberate speed will not take appropriate action to reverse your heartless historicity?[9]

While one may have some sympathy with this view, it is difficult to escape the conclusion as to illegitimacy in any jurisdiction in which legitimacy is conditional upon the existence of a valid subsisting marriage between the parents at the time of conception. The same writer invites a court to hold that 'a posthumously conceived child is the legitimate child of her and her late husband, at least if she has not remarried at the time of conception'. If the woman had remarried at the time of conception there would be a presumption that her new husband was the father of the child. But to take the writer's argument to its logical conclusion, there does not seem to be any reason why the remarriage should make any difference to the child's status. The subsequent marriage would do no more than provide a social father for the child and raise the inference in law that the new husband was the father. It would however be possible to demonstrate that he was not the father and that would raise the question of what status one gives to a child conceived by a woman with the semen of her first husband after his death, but while she was married to someone else.

The second issue which arises relates to the administration of the husband's estate. (In the following discussion this includes the administration of the estate of a cohabitee.) In deciding how the estate of the deceased husband ought to be wound up it may be irrelevant whether the child is regarded as a legitimate child or an illegitimate child. Many jurisdictions confer succession rights on illegitimate children and so any illegitimate children, whenever conceived, might have a right to succeed to their father's estate.

The basic problem is that an estate is generally wound up with reference to the position at the date of death. At that point, all the beneficiaries will generally be known. The only exception is the child conceived prior to, but not born until after, the death. Probably most jurisdictions recognize the right of such children to share in the estate. A child conceived after death will have a right to succeed to the deceased's estate if it is a legitimate child and may in some jurisdictions have a similar right even though it is illegitimate. The problem is that if a person's semen has been stored, his estate could not be wound up until his partner was unable to bear further children or until such time as the semen had been used up.[10] The younger the woman is, the more likely it would be that she could have further children and the greater the interval between the date of death and the final winding up of the estate. While it is improbable that a woman would continue to have, or indeed start to have, children by her partner after his death, the fact that it can be done, and has been done, means that the legal and other issues must be faced. The problem is perhaps more acute where the couple already have children. The central question then becomes how to balance the interests of the children conceived before death with those conceived afterwards.

It would be inequitable to deprive children conceived after death of all rights in their father's estate. It could, however, create serious and perhaps insurmountable problems if a woman had an unfettered right to conceive children after her partner's death. Any time limit which is imposed must be arbitrary. That of itself, however, is no objection to drawing a line at some point, given that there are many other instances in which the law does this. One possibility would be to allow a woman one year after the death in which to conceive a child by her partner, and give the child full succession rights. There are several reasons why the line could be drawn at this point.

A child so conceived would be born within a relatively short time of the death and would not be very much younger than a child conceived immediately before death – this might reduce any social stigma. The interval is sufficiently lengthy to allow the woman time to adjust to the death and consider the implications of posthumous conception for herself, her existing children and the child(ren) to be. Thirdly, the interval would not interfere unduly with the administration of the estate. Some estates take a considerable time to wind up and some of the administration could proceed during this interval. As far as is known, no legislature has yet dealt specifically with this issue.[11] It would not be necessary in any jurisdiction which did not permit succession by illegitimate children, but it would be necessary in all other cases.

The issues just discussed would arise also in connection with egg donation and embryo donation. There is however another matter which arises particularly in relation to embryo donation. At the moment it is not clear in law whether human semen, eggs and embryos are items of property which can be gifted or sold, but there does not seem to be anything to prevent this. That being so, it is theoretically possible for a man to donate his frozen semen, or dispose of it by will. A woman may do likewise with her eggs and a couple may do so with their embryo. There would therefore be nothing to prevent a man giving semen, or a woman giving an egg, to one of their children, and a couple might donate an embryo to their child. If a man gifted semen to his son, the son's wife could be artificially inseminated with it and produce a child whose biological father was also his grandfather, and who would be a half-brother of his mother's husband. If a couple donated an embryo to their son, whose wife had it implanted in her, the subsequent child's grandfather would be its genetic father and its grandmother, the genetic mother. The woman who gave birth to it would be the nurturing mother and she would be obliged to register it as her child. The law has yet to decide whether the genetic mother or the nurturing mother is legally the mother, and so the nurturing mother might also be regarded in law as the mother, especially as she would bring the child up as her own. Her husband would be the child's half-brother but would be presumed in law to be the father, because his wife gave birth to it, and would be regarded as the father by anyone who was unaware of the child's true origins. The child would therefore have two sets of parents and that would naturally create problems for those winding up the estates of the 'grandparents'. While it is unlikely that this would ever be done, there is a need to regulate the use and disposal of human semen, eggs and embryos both during the lifetime of the donor or donors, and also after death.

Confused artificial insemination

In the preceding chapters only two types of artificial insemination have been mentioned, namely artificial insemination using the husband's semen (AIH) and artificial insemination using the semen from a donor (AID). There are however other possibilities, one of which is to use a mixture of the husband's semen and donor semen (AIHD). This is sometimes also called confused artificial insemination (CAI) or mixed artificial insemination (AIM). While some doctors are of the opinion that it is unwise to use such a mixture because it reduces the chances of success,[12] others do not share that view.[13] It is difficult to know how prevalent the use of CAI is, but the principal reason for adopting this method of artificial insemination is to make it more difficult to prove that the husband is *not* the father, or to persuade him more easily that he is.

The legal issues which arise in connection with AIH and AID arise also with CAI, but they are complicated by the fact of the mixing of the semen.

Equally the semen from several donors may be mixed. This may also be known as CAI or AIM. This practice also makes it difficult to establish the identity of the natural father, but it does not give rise to any problems in addition to those which arise from AID.

PART III
EGG DONATION, *IN VITRO* FERTILIZATION, EMBRYO TRANSFER AND DONATION, SURROGACY

13 Donation methods and IVF

Having dealt with the methods of overcoming male infertility it is now appropriate to consider female infertility. In this chapter a number of separate but related treatments will be considered. These are egg donation, which is comparable with AID; *in vitro* fertilization and embryo replacement, which involves fertilization of the egg in laboratory conditions and its replacement into the womb of the person who produced the egg; and it would of course be possible to put the fertilized egg into another woman, which is examined under the heading 'Embryo transfer and donation'.

Egg donation

Where a husband cannot father a child, or there is some reason why he should not do so, AID is one possibility open to the couple. Where the problem lies, not with the man but with the woman, for example where she is unable to ovulate or may pass on some disorder to her natural children, egg donation might be considered. This is an exact counterpart of AID. An egg could be obtained from another woman and fertilized by semen from the first woman's husband, and the fertilized egg would be implanted in the first woman.

Because the process is similar to AID, the only legal issue of any great significance would be the status of the child which is born as the result. Because the child is biologically related to the egg donor and the husband, it is strictly speaking illegitimate. It would however be even more difficult to establish this than in AID, since the woman would give birth to the child and she could register it as her child and her husband's without infringing the relevant legislation. If the identity of the egg donor was kept secret, there would not be any contest between the 'mothers'. If on the other hand, the identity was revealed, which is unlikely, and there was a claim by both 'mothers', a court would have to decide which was to be preferred and why. This problem would arise also in surrogacy and the issues are dealt with in that connection.

In order to avoid any possible dispute about the status of the child, legislation could be enacted along the same lines as that suggested in respect of AID. It would therefore provide that where a married woman, with the consent of her husband, is artificially implanted with an egg from another woman the resulting child should be deemed to be the legitimate child of the first woman and her husband.

In their *Report on In Vitro Fertilisation and Embryo Replacement or Transfer*, the RCOG recommended that an egg donor should surrender all interests in her egg, in the same way as semen donors do in relation to their semen, under the USA legislation.[1] It has also been suggested that egg donation should be permitted under similar safeguards to those governing AID.[2] Egg donation raises issues of maintenance, succession and confidentiality, which have been discussed in the context of AID. There is no UK legislation dealing with the status of children born following egg donation, but the matter has been made more urgent by the announcement in July 1986 of a birth of a child from an egg which had been frozen.[3]

In vitro fertilization and embryo replacement

The birth of Louise Brown – the world's first 'test-tube' baby – at Oldham in July 1978 was the event which brought *in vitro* fertilization (IVF) to the attention of the public. Her birth was the successful outcome of years of work by Dr Robert Edwards and Mr Patrick Steptoe, as narrated in their book *A Matter of Life*, published in 1980.[4]

IVF is a method by which an egg is fertilized under laboratory conditions. After the resulting embryo has developed for a short while it is then replaced into the uterus of the woman who produced the egg. Strictly IVF is the first process only, but for convenience in this chapter 'IVF' is used to cover both processes, unless the context indicates otherwise. More recently French researchers have pioneered a method of injecting sperm into the abdomen where it seems to have a greater chance of fertilizing eggs[5].

IVF can be used where the male is oligospermic and in cases of unexplained infertility. It may also be used where a blockage in the Fallopian tubes prevents sperm and egg meeting. Such a blockage may be caused by disease, or by a sterilization operation. Before a woman with blocked tubes can become pregnant the tubes must be unblocked, or the blockage must be overcome by other means. For example the tubes could be rejoined by surgery, or Fallopian tubes could be transplanted from another woman.[6] IVF is an alternative to these – the egg is removed and is fertilized outside the woman's body and then replaced. While IVF began as an alternative to tubal surgery, it is increasingly used in cases where the infertility is unexplained.[7]

On one analysis of IVF it merely achieves in the laboratory what is otherwise achieved by natural conception. It would be tempting, but wrong, to conclude that the process does not give rise to any legal issues. In the USA considerable thought has been given to the constitutional issues raised by this practice, and something will be said of these later.

However there are legal issues which are perhaps of more immediate concern to the patient and the IVF team. As in other medical procedures, the doctor must obtain the patient's consent and one of the factors which ought to be drawn to her attention is that success cannot be guaranteed even although many children have been born after the thawing of an embryo,[8] and now from an egg which had been frozen.[9] If consent is not obtained the procedure may amount to an assault, or an action based on negligence may be raised if the patient was not given as much information as ought to have been given.[10]

Apart from an action arising out of 'consent', claims might be made by the child or the parents or both, arising from the recovery of the eggs for fertilization, or the process of fertilization and replacement.

Recovery of the egg and replacement of the fertilized embryo

Before fertilization can take place an egg has to be removed from the ovary. It may be located by a surgical procedure known as laparoscopy, or by ultrasound scanning, and thereafter removed. Of the two, ultrasound involves less risk to the patient, but it is not always possible to use this procedure. Once the egg has been fertilized the resulting embryo has to be replaced. This is done by a catheter, which is both safe and simple.

In either process injury may be caused to the woman, or to the egg or embryo, and such an injury could give rise to a claim for damages. This is, however, unlikely.

Achieving fertilization and the development of the embryo

Once the egg has been removed it is fertilized and the subsequent embryo is allowed to develop. In May 1983 Dr Edwards, writing in

Nature, stated that there was a considerable risk of chromosomal damages in human embryos produced by IVF, but in his opinion this could be attributed to technical inadequacies.[11] Once again claims might be made by the child or the parents, especially if it was suggested that a defect in the child could be attributed to such inadequacies.

Action by the child

A legal action by the child could be based on negligence or 'wrongful life'.

Negligence   A claim based on negligence might be raised by a child if it was born with some physical or mental defect. To succeed, the child would have to prove that the defect was caused by the way in which the IVF was carried out, namely that it had not been carried out with the degree of skill which a reasonably competent person in that field would demonstrate.

   An action based on antenatal injuries is recognized in the UK and USA and in a number of other countries.[12] In the USA some jurisdictions tended to adhere to the view that the child must have been viable at the time the injury was caused,[13] but the modern trend is to allow the child to recover from injuries sustained prior to viability.[14] However the child must subsequently be born alive. Claims made by children conceived by IVF will be based on damage done at the embryonic stage – well before viability. The child would have to prove that the injuries arose from the IVF or the replacement, and this might be difficult because many abnormalities do not have an identifiable cause.

Wrongful life   Another possible action is for wrongful life, in which the child claims, not in respect of defects arising from alleged negligence, but in respect of the birth itself. The claim, in essence, is that but for the negligence the child would not have been born – non-existence being preferable to a life of severe handicap. A claim for wrongful life has been raised in the USA by an illegitimate child who argued that to be born illegitimate was disadvantageous,[15] and by a child born to a mentally-deficient woman.[16] In the USA these claims were originally unsuccessful, but recently the courts have looked more favourably on them.[17] In England an action raised by a child which was born handicapped because its mother had contracted German measles during pregnancy was not successful, because the claim was based on wrongful life. The court pointed out that it could not assess the loss to the child on the basis that its existence had not been terminated prior to birth.[18]

A claim based on wrongful life could arise from IVF where, for example, the egg or embryo had been damaged in some way but this had not been noticed, or the damage had not been drawn to the attention of the patient to allow her to decide whether to take the risk of re-implantation, or to try again. The claim would be that if the damage been spotted or the patient advised, the child would not have been born handicapped because it would not have been born at all.

IVF can be used to determine the sex of embryos. This means that by selecting an embryo or embryos of one sex rather than the other, certain genetic diseases can be eliminated, or their incidence reduced. If those performing IVF failed to make the correct decision as to the sex of the embryo which ought to be replaced a child could be born with a disorder, whereas had the correct choice been made it would probably not have been born at all. However, as has been said, the English courts have rejected the only claim which has been made on this basis.

Action by the parents

On the analogy of the child's action for wrongful life, the parents may have an action for wrongful life, the basis being that, had they been properly advised about the risks of having a deformed child, they would have avoided conception or would have destroyed the embryo or terminated the pregnancy. In both the USA[19] and the UK[20] such actions have been held to be competent.

In one US case parents successfully sued in respect of the destruction of a fertilized egg prior to implantation.[21] Dr and Mrs Del Zio claimed $1.5 million in damages from a Manhattan hospital and the doctor, Raymond Vande Wiele. In 1972 Mrs Del Zio agreed to allow Dr Landrum Shettles to proceed with *in vitro* fertilization using her husband's semen. After fertilization, but before implantation, the specimen was destroyed by Dr Vande Wiele, without authority from the Del Zios. Vande Wiele claimed that Dr Shettles lacked the expertise to perform the procedure and that the appropriate hospital committee had not given its approval. Mrs Del Zio claimed that the destruction of the fertilized egg denied her the chance of having a child, and that this caused her physical damage and emotional distress. She was awarded $50,000 and her husband nominal damages. However the action was based not on wrongful destruction of a foetus, but on a loss analogous to property loss. There would not seem to be any doubt that such an action would also succeed in the UK, on the analogy that actions have succeeded in the UK where a child has been born after an unsuccessful sterilization.[22] If the destruction of an embryo without consent gives rise to claim for damages, it would seem that actions could equally succeed in respect of the unauthorized destruction of sperm or eggs.

Surplus embryos

Until now, reference has been made to the recovery of one egg and the creation of one embryo. At a fairly early stage in IVF it was realized that there was a greater chance of a pregnancy if more than one embryo was reimplanted.[23] The voluntary licensing authority has recommended that not more than three embryos should be reimplanted.[24] The possibility of creating more than one embryo arises from the use of superovulatory drugs, which result in a number of eggs, all of which can be fertilized.

The creation of a number of embryos with a view to reimplanting some, but not all, of them raises the important issue of the status of the embryo. This arises acutely in connection with surplus or spare embryos, but it arises automatically from the creation of even one embryo. If that embryo fails to develop properly, can the IVF team decide not to reimplant it, or is it protected because the union of sperm and egg has created a human being or a potential human being? This is essentially an ethical issue, but the law ought to pronounce upon it sooner rather than later. In order to ascertain the current legal position of the embryo it is useful to consider first the status of human semen and human eggs.

Legal status of semen and eggs   The human body occupies a unique position in law. It is not a piece of property[25] and, in the absence of statutory authority such as that on anatomical donation, a person cannot contract for the sale of his body or parts of it, nor can he give them away during his lifetime or bequeath them in his will.

Obvious exceptions to this are donations of blood, semen and eggs. These can be regarded as the provision of a service rather than the sale of a product. This issue has not come before the courts in the UK, but, as was noted earlier, this has been the approach in courts in the USA when they considered it in connection with the blood transfusion service. Over forty states now have legislation which recognizes that the provision of blood is a service rather than a sale.[26] Sperm and eggs can also be regenerated and, even though the former is frequently supplied for a fee, it is suggested that the correct approach is to regard this as a service rather than a sale.

The legal position is probably this. Semen and eggs, like blood, are body products which are items of property but cannot be disposed of at will. They cannot be sold, but may be made available to others as a gift or as a service for which payment may be made. The Draft Recommendations of the Council of Europe take the strict line that semen and eggs are *extra commercium* and that no payment ought to be made in respect of them.[27] The next issue is how the law regards the result of the union of sperm and egg – the embryo.

Legal status of the embryo

Fertilization of the egg produces an embryo which is a new creation, but, unlike either the sperm or the egg, it is not capable of regeneration. The embryo can be identified as human material and, while in most cases it will have a unique genetic structure, this is not so in every case. The embryo may split to produce identical twins,but not later than day 15. What can be said is that if the embryo is left to develop in the mother's womb, a live child or children might result. There is of course no guarantee that this will happen given the high percentage of embryos which fail to implant and the incidence of spontaneous abortions.

The legal issue is not when life begins, but at what point the embryo is recognized in law and acquires rights or is given some protection. Even if the issue was couched in terms of when human life begins, it is not possible to give an unequivocal response.[28] The Roman Catholic Church and others hold that life begins at fertilization[29] but this is not the stance traditionally taken, even by Roman Catholic theologians,[30] and very recently one distinguished theologian has dissented from that view.[31]

In trying to ascertain the legal position it is necessary to look at related areas of law, for there is no legislation or case law which deals specifically or by inference with the status of the embryo. These analogies may be drawn from both the civil and the criminal law.

Civil law   In the USA there has been some litigation arising from hospitals losing or destroying foetuses and the bodies of still-born babies which the parents wanted to bury. These actions were argued on the basis that emotional distress had been caused to the parents, rather than on any other ground such as wrongful disposal of property.[32] In the Del Zio case the jury appears to have rejected the notion that the embryo was a piece of property and awarded damages solely for the distress caused to the parents.

In 1972 a UK committee considered the use of foetal material for research and it stated, somewhat ambiguously, that there was no statutory provision which required the consent of parents for the use of foetal material in research. Equally there was no provision which expressly dispensed with it.[33] From that, it may be accepted that a foetus is not regarded as property, but before it can be regarded as having rights it must be shown to have legal personality.

In that connection it may be argued that a child may claim for ante-natal injury and it may acquire property while it is *in utero*. That, however, does not take the discussion any further because in either case the child does not acquire these rights unless it is born alive. If therefore a child suffers ante-natal injury, no claim can be raised on its behalf if it is aborted or still-born. The same applies to the child's contingent interest in property. There are no other analogies in the field of civil law, and accordingly we pass to the criminal law to see what assistance it affords.

Criminal law   In criminal law the closest analogy is abortion. The US Supreme Court has held that a mother may terminate her pregnancy provided the foetus is not viable, and it observed that the state's interest in protecting potential human life becomes compelling only when a foetus reaches that state which it defined as 'the interim point at which the foetus becomes . . . potentially able to live outside the mother's womb, albeit with artificial aid'.[34]

In both the USA and the UK it has been held that a woman may obtain an abortion without her husband's consent.[35] These decisions suggest that the courts are not prepared to regard a foetus as having legal personality and that it is really a part of the woman, which makes her husband's consent irrelevant.

In the UK an abortion is legal only if it is carried out within the terms of the Abortion Act 1967. If it is not, in England and Wales there may be a contravention of the Offences Against the Person Act 1861, or in Scotland a crime at common law. Recently in England, a complaint was made to the Director of Public Prosecutions about the so-called 'morning after pill'. It was suggested that its use was, in reality, an abortion and therefore an infringement of the 1861 Act. The Act talks about 'procuring a miscarriage' and in a statement to Parliament the Attorney-General said:

> It is clear that, used in its ordinary sense the word 'miscarriage' is not apt to describe a failure to implant, whether spontaneous or not. Likewise the phrase 'procuring a miscarriage' cannot be construed to include the prevention of implantation[36]

That statement is not binding on the courts, but it does mean that the Attorney-General will not prosecute those who use these devices. It would be stretching what was said to argue that he recognized that legal personality did not begin at fertilization, but what is clear is that the fact that an egg has been fertilized is not itself sufficient to entitle it to protection.

Neither the civil nor the criminal law throws much light on the issue, but what guidance there is suggests that the embryo does not have legal personality and would not acquire it until it became capable of existing outside the mother's body. That view finds some support among theologians and philosophers. One eminent Anglican theologian concludes that, historically, the protection given to the foetus increased as it developed, and that the claim to absolute protection from the moment of fertilization is virtually a creation of the later nineteenth century.[37]

Despite what has been said on this issue, whether by scientists, doctors, theologians, lawyers or others, people will continue to have different views. Society has to determine whether protection is to be afforded to the embryo, what form it is to take and when it will begin.

The law could give the embryo full protection at two stages – at fertilization or some later point. Without in any way prejudging the issue, it is quite clear that if the law affords full protection to the embryo at fertilization, IVF probably could not be carried out and it would not be possible to do research on surplus embryos.

IVF could not be carried out because, once the embryos had been created, they would all have to be reimplanted and could not be disposed of even if they were defective. They would be entitled to the full protection given to other human beings, as would embryos deliberately created for research.

If however protection is not given until some later stage, it is clear that in the intervening period some research could be done. It seems that society would in general favour this, but it would wish to have some control over the nature and duration of research. If it is a generally held view that there ought to be some control, the next question is what form the control should take. In this connection, it is instructive to look at what has happened in the UK, the USA and Australia.

United Kingdom

Although the first child conceived by IVF was born in July 1978, it was not until July 1982 that the government announced the setting up of a committee under the chairmanship of Baroness Warnock to examine the various issues raised by this and related practices.[38] In the interval a significant number of IVF children had been born in the UK and elsewhere. However, prior to the announcement, various influential bodies including the RCOG, the MRC, the BMA and the Royal Society had set up their own committees to examine the issues, and many others did so in response to the Warnock Committee. Each one of these bodies recognized the benefits of some form of research on surplus embryos. However, as one might expect, opinions were divided on what kinds of research should be done and for how long.

The Royal Society drew a distinction between embryos obtained for therapeutic purposes and those obtained for research purposes, and it stated that the latter should not be used for reimplantation. However research projects are in its view 'best handled by local ethical committees' and it favoured 'a degree of flexibility' in the regulation of work on human fertilization and embryology.[39]

The MRC gave a clear statement of its views:

Scientifically-sound research involving experiments on the process and products of *in vitro* fertilization between human gametes is ethically acceptable and should be allowed to proceed on condition that there is no intent to transfer to the uterus any embryo resulting from or used in such experiments and also that the aim of the research is clearly defined and directly relevant to clinical problems such as contraception or the differential diagnosis and treatment of infertility and inherited diseases.

However, it went on to say that surplus embryos should not be cultured beyond the implantation stage and should not be stored for unspecified scientific use.[40] The RCOG also took the view that research on human embryos was acceptable and supported the approach of the MRC. However the RCOG was of the opinion that no embryo should be allowed to develop beyond 'the stage of early neural development (Day 17 after conception . . .)'

The RCOG took a different approach from the Royal Society and suggested legislative powers to supervize IVF, these powers to be exercised by the Secretary of State. The legislation should create a register of directors of licensed institutions, but it could not, and should not, attempt to regulate the techniques. In addition a statutory body should be set up to advise the Secretary of State on matters relating to IVF and he would have powers to make regulations following on the advice. The RCOG clearly recognized that society as a whole has an interest in ensuring that IVF is carried out for its benefit and those of the couples and children involved. This could best be done by some form of parliamentary control. Such control could take the form of a highly detailed code dealing with all aspects of the subject, but that could be unduly restrictive. A better approach would be to have overall control vested in Parliament, leaving the daily work to the doctors and scientists with freedom to experiment subject only to the overall control.[41]

Finally the BMA also established a working group which reported in May 1983. It supported experimental work, but concluded that it should not be carried out after the 14th day after fertilization. The BMA group also accepted the statement made by the MRC.[42]

While each of these bodies supported the principle of research on surplus embryos, not everyone shares that view, and a contrary approach can be seen in the evidence submitted to Warnock by the Catholic Bishops' Joint Committee on Bioethical Issues.[43] In their view, all of the following are unacceptable and ought to be prohibited:

(i) any form of experimentation on a human embryo which is likely to damage that human embryo, or endangers it by delaying the time of its transfer and implantation, other than procedures intended to benefit that embryo itself;

(ii) any form of observation of a human embryo which damages that human embryo, or endangers it by delaying the time of its transfer and implantation, other than observations made for the benefit of that embryo itself;

(iii) any form of freezing or other storage done without genuine and definite prospect of subsequent transfer, unimpaired to the proper mother;

(iv) any form of selection among living and developing human embryos, with a view to transferring and implanting only the fittest or most desirable.[44]

The reason for objecting to these practices, the bishops say, is that they 'involve one human being sitting in judgement on the very life of another and treating that other as a mere means to an end (perhaps a very worthy end); or one human being along with a disregard for that other's well-being which amounts to treating that other as a mere means'. Implicit in this is the view that human life begins at fertilization, a point which is made explicitly in the same paper.[45] Similar views are expressed in a Vatican pronouncement in March 1987 which is referred to in the final chapter.

United States

In the USA the Department of Health, Education and Welfare (DHEW) (now the Department of Health and Human Services) funded research into IVF until Congress banned foetal research in July 1974. The ban was lifted in August 1975 when the DHEW promulgated regulations requiring all proposals seeking funds for foetal research to be reviewed by a national Ethics Advisory Board (EAB).

After the birth of Louise Brown, the EAB was instructed in September 1978 to consider the social, legal, ethical and medical implications of a particular research project. However, it was also to conduct public hearings on IVF in general. It examined the subject and presented its final report in May 1979. The board concluded that IVF research and embryo transfer was 'acceptable from an ethical standpoint', and that research on pre-implantation embryos was ethical, provided it would further knowledge about the clinical applications of IVF. The board had this to say: '[T]he human embryo is entitled to profound respect, but this respect does not necessarily encompass the full legal and moral rights attributed to a person . . . some embryo loss associated with attempts to assist otherwise infertile couples through *in vitro* fertilization may be regarded as acceptable from an ethical standpoint under certain conditions.'[46] The board's findings were made public in June 1979 and about 13 000 comments were received – the majority negative, as was the response from Congress. The *de facto* moratorium remains because successive Secretaries of the Department have not accepted the board's findings. There does not seem to be any doubt that most scientists would favour the ending of the moratorium, but it remains to be seen whether this will happen.[47]

Australia

Even before the birth of Louise Brown in 1978, the Australian Law Reform Committee had indicated that there was a need to examine the whole area of IVF.[48] However a new Attorney-General was firmly of the view that laws dealing with IVF were a matter for individual states rather than the federal government. Inquiries were instituted in all the states, but only in New South Wales and Victoria has there been any legislation.[49] The inquiry set up in Victoria reported in August 1983 and it made these recommendations:

(a) the use of donor semen and eggs should be permitted;
(b) comprehensive information ought to be made available to infertile couples;
(c) that counselling should precede, accompany and follow participation where couples want to take part in IVF with donated sperm and/or eggs;
(d) that the written consent of sperm and egg donors should be obtained;
(e) that donors should not be paid;
(f) that the use of known donors should be permitted where both 'parents' desire;
(g) that subject to (f) donors should be anonymous but that couples should be given information, for example about physical characteristics, if they wished.

IVF has progressed a great deal in Australia, but it is open to serious doubt whether all the states will issue reports and implement them in legislation which will be identical. The developments in Australia are discussed again in the final chapter.

It remains to be seen what will be the full results of these various deliberations on research on human embryos, but any legislation, or any other consideration of IVF, will need to decide on the status of the embryo, and hence that of surplus embryos. The legislation in Victoria does so.

If the view is that life begins at fertilization it follows that all embryos, including those which are left over from one attempt at implantation, must be implanted, as they are human beings or potential human beings. If however the embryo is not given legal status until later, it will nevertheless be important to have provisions regulating its use prior to the time at which protection is afforded.

At present in the UK many clinics will have a number of surplus or spare embryos. If no special provisions govern these, they are either human beings or items of property. It is therefore desirable that legislation, which confers legal status on embryos at some time after fertilization, should also prevent embryos being sold by the couples who created them or by the clinics, and also prevent them being used by governments as part of any 'selective breeding programme'.

As the law stands in the UK, the USA and any other countries where there is no specific legislation on the subject, there seems to be nothing which would prevent embryos being sold, gifted or otherwise disposed of at will.

Embryo transfer and donation

At one time the term 'embryo transfer' was used to describe the replacement of the fertilized egg after IVF. The 'transfer' would be into the uterus of the woman who produced the egg. 'Embryo transfer' is not appropriate to describe this[50] and the term 'embryo replacement' is now used to cover what was previously known as embryo transfer.[51]

'Embryo transfer' or 'embryo donation' describes the situation in which the fertilized egg is implanted into another woman. There is however a distinction to be drawn between embryo transfer and embryo donation. In embryo donation the intention is that the embryo is given to the other woman and that she will be the child's mother for all purposes. It is therefore analogous to sperm donation or egg donation.

Embryo transfer is a wider term. While it covers the situation in which the implanted embryo is donated to the other woman, it can also describe the case where the other woman is merely to carry the embryo until birth and then hand the child back to the genetic parents – the donors. It is then an element in a surrogacy arrangement, which is dealt with in Chapter 14.

When the embryo is produced its genetic parents are of course the donors of the sperm and egg. The embryo has no genetic link with the gestational mother, nor will it have any link with her husband. If her husband had provided the semen, this is egg donation, not embryo donation.

One of the legal problems which arises from embryo donation, as with egg donation, is that the child would have two 'mothers'. The implications of this have already been dealt with, and it was noted that UK law has yet to decide which is the mother – the woman who produces the egg or the woman who gives birth to the child.

The child might also have two 'fathers' – the genetic father who produced the sperm and the husband of the woman who gave birth to the child, the 'social' father. The donor of the sperm need not be married to the donor of the egg.

A contest between the mothers or the fathers, or a dispute about the legal position of the child *vis-à-vis* its social father is not likely to arise if embryo donation, like AID, is done anonymously.

If however the child's origins were disclosed, it would be in the same position as regards the social father as an AID child, and in the same position as regards the gestational mother as a child born as the result of egg donation.

To resolve these issues where the embryo is truly donated, UK law should provide that the gestational mother and her husband are deemed to be the father and mother of the child for all purposes and that the donors have no rights in the child, nor it in them.

The other issues raised by embryo donation are dealt with in the earlier chapters on AID.

14 Surrogacy

In the last few years a considerable amount of publicity has been given to infertile couples who have agreed with another woman that she will carry a child for them and hand it over to them after its birth. This practice has been described in various ways, such as 'womb-leasing', or 'hostess mothering'. Throughout this book however the word 'surrogacy' is used because it is less emotive than 'womb-leasing' and is the term now most frequently used to describe the arrangement. Some authors have attempted to draw a distinction between 'womb-leasing' and surrogacy,[1] but no such distinction is drawn here and it is questionable whether any such distinction is useful or necessary.

Having said that, it is important to define the term 'surrogacy' as covering any situation in which one woman agrees to carry a child for another. This includes a case where a couple decide to hand over their child to another couple; also an arrangement whereby a woman is artificially inseminated with semen by a man who, with his wife or partner, will be the child's 'parents'; and finally a situation in which a woman has another couple's embryo implanted in her, on the understanding that she will surrender the child to the couple who produced the embryo, or possibly to someone else. The possible permutations are shown in the Appendix.

Agreements to have children by surrogates may be attractive for several reasons. For example, a couple may not be able to have children because the woman is infertile or there are medical reasons why she should not have children. There is of course the possibility of adoption, but apart from the shortage of children available for adoption, there are other reasons why this might not be an alternative. The couple may have been trying for a number of years to have children; they will probably be older and perhaps regarded as less suitable candidates. Some couples may not consider adoption because of the fear of rejection by society or because of their social or financial position. The child who is adopted will have no genetic links with the adopting parents, whereas a child born to a surrogate will, in many cases, be the child of one of the couple – usually the man. Some couples might consider using a surrogate where the woman is pursuing a career which would be adversely affected by pregnancy. If the current trend towards careers for married women continues, surrogacy may have an increasing appeal.

In a recent book[2] the authors give helpful descriptions of the various women involved. These help to clarify their roles, but also aid the understanding of the legal links with the child. They mention three categories of mother: the genetic mother, the carrying mother and the nurturing mother; and the possible permutations, namely complete mother, genetic-carrying mother, genetic-nurturing mother, nurturing-carrying mother.

The genetic mother is the woman who produces the egg. The authors prefer this term to 'biological mother' which, in their view, could cover the woman who carries the child whom they describe as the 'carrying mother'. The nurturing mother is the woman who will look after the child once it is born. These descriptions are most helpful and are therefore used throughout this chapter.

It can readily be appreciated that surrogacy may involve artificial insemination, egg donation or embryo transfer. Equally, however, it need not involve any of them and for that reason it may be suggested that a discussion of surrogacy has no place in a book dealing with artificial reproduction. The main reasons for including it are that the instances so far *have* involved artificial insemination and that, considered from the standpoint of the intended nurturing parents, it is an artificial method of having a child.

History of surrogacy

Surrogacy has received publicity since the late 1970s and it has frequently been assumed that the practice is a recent development. However there are two biblical passages which can be construed as examples of surrogacy,[3] and it would be rash to assume that surrogacy was never practised prior to the 1970s. While it is impossible to say how old the practice is, in so far as it involves artificial insemination it is recent, as is its organization on a commercial basis.

The surrogacy agreements which have received publicity so far have involved an infertile wife whose husband has artificially inseminated another woman who has agreed to hand over the child to the couple after its birth, with the intention that the couple should adopt it. In most cases the surrogate has agreed to do this only for a fee, but there have been a few cases, for example where

the women were related, in which there was no financial consideration. In all cases the important element was the agreement by the
carrying mother to surrender the child to the nurturing mother and
her partner.

Usually it is a married couple who enter into the arrangement
and the surrogate will almost invariably receive payment or its
equivalent. It is assumed here that this is so, unless the context
indicates otherwise.

Most recently attention has focused on surrogacy agreements
because American agencies have been set up in the UK. They
charge a fee to the couple, some of which is paid to the surrogate.
The nurturing mother and her partner enter into a formal written
agreement with the agency, as does the surrogate. Clearly the
practice of surrogacy, especially on a commercial basis, raises a
number of ethical, social and legal issues, but this chapter deals
almost exclusively with the latter.

Is surrogacy the same as baby-buying?

The first legal issue is whether surrogacy is struck at because it is,
in reality, baby-buying. This question has been considered in the
USA but not in the UK, although in both countries children are not
regarded as items of property. In the USA, the practice of baby-
buying, which occurred frequently with Vietnamese children, has
been the subject of scrutiny by the Sub-Committee on Children and
Youth of the Committee on Labor and Welfare.[4] This investigation
was prompted by the activities of certain US attorneys, one of
whom, Ronald Silverton, was indicted on fourteen charges of
criminal conspiracy and related contraventions of the adoption
legislation. The sub-committee heard evidence that there were
about 5000 such arrangements in the USA every year, and that
substantial sums were paid to mothers to surrender their children.[5]
In the course of the evidence it was noted that some attorneys who
were involved paid women to become pregnant in order to keep
up with demand.[6] The Attorney-General of New York expressed
an opinion in 1975 that this arrangement infringed the law which
prohibited private placements for adoption.

It seems that in the USA and the UK baby-buying can take place
only where there is a live child. It is therefore distinguishable from
surrogacy where the woman is paid to become pregnant and carry
a child. While surrogacy arrangements may not therefore amount
to baby-buying, there may be other legal objections to the practice.

United States constitutional issues

Another issue which has been discussed in the USA, but would not arise in the UK, is whether a person has a constitutional right to be a surrogate mother or to employ such a person. Putting the point slightly differently, the issue is whether prohibition of surrogacy arrangements would be an infringement of the constitutional right of privacy. That would be an issue for the federal courts, and ultimately the US Supreme Court, to decide. However, while there might be an infringement of privacy, a court may consider other factors, such as those which persuaded the UK government to ban commercial surrogacy.[7]

In discussions of this issue some reference has been made to the Universal Declaration of Human Rights (1948) and the European Convention on Human Rights (1953). Article 16(1) of the Universal Declaration of Human Rights says: 'Men and women of full age . . . have the right to marry and to found a family.' Article 12 of the European Convention on Human Rights is in similar terms: 'Men and women of marriageable age have the right to marry and to found a family.'

In the USA the regulation of domestic relations was regarded at one time as being solely within the province of state law.[8] Recently, however, state legislation has been more subject to federal scrutiny and limitations because of this constitutional right of privacy.[9] It has been held that there are areas in which the state should not interfere without justification. These include decisions about whether or not to marry,[10] to have children,[11] to practise contraception[12] or have an abortion.[13] It might be argued that a statute which directly or indirectly prohibits surrogacy infringes the right of privacy, since it would interfere with the freedom to have a family. However, even if that was accepted, it would not, of itself, render the statute invalid, as the interference by the state may be justifiable. In most instances the state does not interfere, partly because of the right to privacy, but also because interference is usually unnecessary, in that the parental desire to have children and the existence of blood ties will normally ensure that the children's interests are protected.[14]

Having said that, there are areas where the state does intervene to protect children, the most notable being adoption. There are several reasons for this. The child does not have a blood tie with both adoptive parents and, in many cases, it does not have a blood tie with either parent. Furthermore it may be argued that if the adopting mother has not experienced the psychological effects of pregnancy and childbirth, it cannot be assumed that she and her partner will further the child's interests in the same way as natural parents. Most important of all, perhaps, is the fact that if the adoption is not successful the state will have the responsibility for looking after the child. That in itself justifies its being involved in the adoption process.

In a surrogacy arrangement the carrying mother will not be the same person as the nurturing mother, and it usually contemplates that the nurturing mother and her partner will adopt the child in order to sever any legal ties which the carrying mother may have.

The state might therefore attempt to control or prohibit surrogacy if it conflicts with the letter or the spirit of the adoption legislation. In a recent case a statute outlawing black market adoptions was challenged by a couple on the ground that it was unconstitutional. They wished to have a child under a surrogacy arrangement. Their argument was rejected for two reasons – that there is no fundamental right to adopt a child, and that the prospective adopters could not invoke the state adoption machinery for one purpose, but reject it for others.[15] If that decision is correct, and in the author's view it is, adoption legislation cannot be challenged as unconstitutional because it might outlaw surrogacy arrangements.

While the issue of constitutionality would not arise in the UK because of the different legal system, it might be argued that any common law or statutory provision within the UK which prohibited or restricted surrogacy was an infringement of the European Convention on Human Rights. This would not be a matter for the UK courts to decide, but for the European Commission, and ultimately the European Court of Human Rights. Apart from the issue of constitutionality, there are other important legal issues. The first is whether it is a criminal offence to enter into a surrogacy agreement, and the second whether the civil courts would enforce such agreements, even if they did not infringe the criminal law.

Criminal law

In the UK there is legislation which prohibits surrogacy on a commerical basis, and such an agreement is also likely to infringe the criminal law if it contravenes the adoption legislation. As has been said, one common feature of surrogacy is that the carrying mother receives a payment or other valuable consideration for her services. (In March 1986 the West German government announced its intention to ban commerical surrogacy.)[16]

In the UK[17] (and many other jurisdictions) there are express provisions in the adoption legislation about payments. They prohibit payments or rewards:

(a)   in order to adopt child;

(b)   to obtain any necessary consent;
(c)   for the transfer of a child with a view to its being adopted;
(d)   for making arrangements for an adoption.

The legislation does not prohibit payments being made to an adoption society or a local authority, provided the payment is to cover reasonable expenses. Similar provisions exist in the USA,[18] for example in California,[19] Michigan,[20] Illinois,[21] New Jersey;[22] and in the Uniform Adoptive Placement Act.[23]

It has been said of these provisions that they are rarely enforced,[24] and there are no reported cases in the UK. Nevertheless their existence constitutes an apparent threat to any surrogacy arrangement which contemplates payment or reward; but before concluding that that apparent threat is also real, it is necessary to examine these provisions more closely.

Adoption Legislation

The first thing that should be said about the adoption statutes is that one object is to prohibit the sale of children as though they were items of property.[25] Children are not the property of their parents and cannot be the subject of a commercial transaction.[26] What appears to be struck at primarily is the sale of illegitimate children by mothers whose pregnancies were unwanted. Many such mothers might wish to keep their children but would not be able to support them. An arrangement whereby someone else 'bought' such a child might therefore have considerable appeal. The purchasers may not wish the transaction to be scrutinized and so would try to avoid the application of the adoption legislation. If they succeed, the arrangement will not be the subject of any enquiry, the prospective parents will escape evaluation and the child's interests – which are of paramount importance in adoption[27] – will not be considered. Furthermore the mother may experience acute distress and guilt at parting with the child without having an opportunity of changing her mind before matters are finalized.[28]

Most surrogacy arrangements will probably contravene the spirit and the letter of the adoption legislation, in that they will usually involve a payment to the carrier and she would probably not be given an opportunity to keep the child if she wished to. However, the adoption legislation does not distinguish between the genetic mother and the carrier. Where the genetic mother and the carrier are the same, the adoption legislation allows her a period in which to consider whether she wishes to give the child up. It is not clear whether this right applies to the carrier where she is not genetically-linked with the child, as would be the case where an embryo was implanted into the carrier.

It could be argued that the reasoning behind the adoption legislation – to protect those whose pregnancies have not been planned – does not apply to surrogacy where the carrier has made a conscious decision to become pregnant and has undertaken to surrender the child. If that argument does not succeed the prohibition against making payment or giving rewards for adoption remains and there would have to be other arguments for taking surrogacy outwith the legislation on adoption.

It might be suggested that the payment in surrogacy is made to the surrogate for agreeing to carry the child, and so is compensation for the pregnancy. The adoption legislation does not make it a crime for someone to become pregnant. The difficulty is that the surrogate hands over the child and receives payment for doing so, and she knows that the couple will have to adopt the child if they wish to have full legal ties with it. It is therefore difficult to divorce the adoption from the payment, even though the adoption of the child is only one of the objects of surrogacy.

Another approach is to say either that the ambit of the adoption legislation is in doubt or that the language used is not clear, and so the legislation ought to be strictly construed, which is the usual approach to legislation which imposes penal sanctions.[29] On the other hand if there is doubt about the meaning or extent of legislative provisions the courts might give effect to the purpose of the statute rather than interpret it strictly if that would give rise to either an absurdity or injustice.[30]

However appealing the arguments for suggesting that surrogacy agreements do not infringe the adoption legislation, it is thought that the courts would probably take the view that the object of the agreement is that one woman should surrender the child and her legal rights and obligations after its birth. In the arrangements which have been discussed recently the surrogate has been the genetic mother and so, in law, she would be the child's natural mother. As the law stands the only way in which she could surrender her rights to another couple would be by adoption. The adoption legislation is designed to secure the best interests of the child by having some scrutiny of intending adopters, and at the same time allowing the natural mother to keep her child if she so desires.

Surrogacy agreements do not necessarily have the best interests of the child in mind, but even if they do they would not envisage that the surrogate could keep the child if she wished, nor would they contemplate any scrutiny of the intended nurturing couple by the state authorities. For these reasons surrogacy arrangements probably infringe the adoption legislation and would certainly do so if a payment, or its equivalent, was given to the surrogate, which will usually be the case.

However, in the only case thus far, in the UK, Latey J. decided that in the particular case, the payment made in respect of a surrogacy arrangement did not infringe the adoption legislation.[31] In that case, a couple, Mr & Mrs A sought to adopt a child which had been born following a surrogacy arrangement. Mrs B was the natural mother and the child had been conceived as the result of sexual intercourse between Mr A and Mrs B, the surrogate. The reason for the surrogacy arrangement was that Mrs A was unable to bear a child; she and her husband had tried to adopt a child both here and abroad, but without success. Mr and Mrs A paid the surrogate a total of £5,000, but she declined a further payment of £5,000. The court held firstly that the money had been paid for the surrogacy and that it was only after the birth of the child that Mr and Mrs A began to think about adoption. For that reason, the payment did not contravene the Adoption Act 1958.[32] However, the judge went on to hold that, even if that was incorrect, the relevant section of the Act[33] excluded 'any payment or reward authorized by the court.' He decided that a court could authorize a payment after the event and in the particular case, he would authorize such a payment.

Surrogacy Arrangements Act 1985

Some of the issues arising from surrogacy were highlighted in January 1985 with the birth of Baby Cotton, whose mother had been employed by an English surrogacy agency which is linked with Surrogate Parenting Inc. of the USA.[34] She entered into a commercial arrangement and agreed to hand the child over when it was born. After the birth the local authority wanted to take the child into care, but it was made a ward of court and the High Court was asked to decide the issue of custody. It was awarded to the natural father and he was given permission to take the child abroad, which he did. In making this decision the court took the correct approach in trying to reach a decision which was in the best interests of the child.

However, because of the publicity surrounding the case and the involvement of a commercial agency, the government introduced legislation – the Surrogacy Arrangements Act 1985 – which outlaws commercial surrogacy and bans advertising about it. The Act reflects the thinking of the Warnock Committee, but there have already been attempts to get round it by paying surrogates for keeping diaries of their pregnancies.[35] The Act deals only with commercial surrogacy, but a Private Member's Bill which was introduced in

November 1985 and sought to extend the provisions of the Act to all surrogacy arrangements failed.

Registration of births

If embryo transfer has taken place the birth should be registered by the gestational mother. In the UK the obligation to register a birth rests primarily with the parents,[36] but the registration should show the surrogate as the mother. If she did not register the child as hers she would be committing a criminal offence.

In the area of criminal law therefore, surrogacy agreements may infringe the adoption legislation and the Surrogacy Arrangement Act 1985, and the nurturing couple might be guilty of a criminal offence if they registered the child as theirs. The surrogate may also commit a criminal offence if she fails to register the child as hers.

Consideration will now be given to the civil law implications of a surrogacy arrangement.

Civil law

Contract

The issue here is whether a surrogacy agreement will be enforced by the courts. There are really three questions: whether there is a contract; whether the contract is enforceable; and assuming the contract is enforceable how it can be enforced.

Is there a contract?   In Anglo-American jurisdictions, but not in Scots law, the existence of a contract is dependent upon 'consideration'.[37] In common parlance consideration is cash or some valuable equivalent, but in law the doctrine is complex and need not be explored here in any detail. What can be said is that if cash or other reward is to be paid to the surrogate this would amount to 'consideration'. Where there is no cash or other reward the position is less certain, but the fact that the surrogate promises to bear the child and to hand it over in exchange for various promises by the couple would probably also amount to consideration.[38] Accordingly even without the financial inducements the arrangement would probably be a contract.

In other jurisdictions which do not require consideration a seriously intended promise may be enforced, as will a definite offer which is met by a definite acceptance.[39] A surrogacy agreement would therefore be a contract.

Is the contract enforceable?   A more important issue is whether the courts will enforce the contract. At this point we must consider whether a contract which infringes the adoption or other legislation, for example the Surrogacy Arrangements Act 1985, may nevertheless be enforced. Equally we must ask whether a surrogacy contract is enforceable, even if it does not contravene that legislation.

Agreement which contravenes the adoption legislation

If the arrangement contravenes some legislation, it might be thought that the civil courts would not enforce the agreement. While this is true in many instances, it is far from being a universal rule.[40] As a general rule the civil courts will look to the intention of legislation to determine whether the contract is struck at.[41]

In most jurisdictions this matter has never arisen in connection with surrogacy, but there have been at least five important cases in the USA. In all of these an agreement was entered into for the adoption of a child and payments were part of the bargain, but the arrangement was not struck down.

In the first case, *In re Shirk*,[42] there was an arrangement between a child's mother and its grandmother, whereby the mother consented to the child being adopted by the grandmother. The child was already in the grandmother's care because the mother was financially incapable of supporting it. In return the grandmother agreed that both the mother and the child would share in her estate on her death. At a later stage the parties agreed to the re-adoption of the child by its mother and her second husband. The issue was the validity of the claims by the mother and the child on the grandmother's estate. The Kansas Supreme Court had to consider whether the contract was against 'good morals and public policy'.

The court was clear that it was 'fundamental that parties may not barter or sell their children, nor may they demand pecuniary gain as the price of consent to adoption'.[43] However, it thought that the arrangement had been entered into to provide the best possible home for the child. Accordingly what it described as a 'family compact' was in the best interests of the child and not contrary to public policy. The court made the following observation:

> [A] contract of a parent by which he bargains away for his pecuniary gain the custody of his child to a stranger and attempts to relieve himself from all parental obligations, placing the burden on another who assumes it, without natural affection or moral obligation, but only because of the bargain, is void as against public policy. Such a contract would be the mere sale of the child for money. But the instant case involves a family compact. The proposal for adoption upon which the

contract was based came from the grandmother. It was not prompted by self-seeking on the part of the mother. Implicit in it is the favourable inference that the controlling consideration was the welfare of the two-year-old child. That fact permeates all the circumstances alleged. While the mother received the promise of the grandmother that she would receive one third of her estate we cannot say that, under all the circumstances alleged and the favourable inferences to which they are entitled, the mother's consent to the adoption falls within the rule that a parent may not transfer his parental rights and duties to another in an attempt to sell or barter his child for his own financial gain.[44]

While there are differences between the circumstances in *Shirk* and those in surrogacy there are also marked similarities. The court in *Shirk* stressed that the arrangement had been suggested, and the initiative taken, by the grandmother who wished to adopt the child, and was not 'prompted by self-seeking on the part of the mother'.[45] That would also be the case in surrogacy where the first steps would be taken by the couple who wanted to have a child, even though the surrogate may have indicated that she was willing to act.

The prime factor in *Shirk* was the welfare of the child. In surrogacy the welfare of the child might arguably be best achieved if it was adopted by the intended parent(s), rather than have it remain with the surrogate, who in all but a few cases will not wish to keep the child. If they were not willing to adopt the child the surrogate would probably place it for adoption elsewhere.

A third point is that, in *Shirk*, the court emphasized 'the family compact'. It could be argued that, in many surrogacy arrangements, there is also a family compact. The only situation in which that would not be the case would be where neither of the intended parents had a genetic link with the child. However, in *Shirk* it was held that both parties had acted out of affection for the child and not for financial reasons. In surrogacy the carrying mother would probably be acting primarily, if not entirely, for gain, but that is not necessarily a fundamental objection, on the analogy of *Shirk*, where the mother ultimately benefited under the grandmother's will.

Given the facts and the decision in *Shirk*, and its similarities to a surrogacy agreement, it is possible to argue that the mere fact that a payment is made by the couple to the surrogate mother is not in itself enough to make the agreement contrary to public policy, nor to imply that it is not in the best interests of the child.

This view is fortified by the decision in another USA case, *Reimche v. First National Bank of Nevada*,[46] which is not dissimilar to *Shirk*. In *Reimche* the agreement was between the natural mother and the father of the child. The mother agreed to consent to adoption by the father who in turn promised to make provision for her and the child in his will. As in *Shirk*, the court distinguished the circumstances from 'baby-buying' principally because the arrangement was between members of a family. It observed: 'The fears that approval of such policy would lead to the bartering or sale of children are not borne out where we deal only with agreements between parents or close family members.'[47] Earlier in its judgment the court had commented on the issue of public policy:

> [I]t is not against public policy to enforce an agreement to provide for the mother of an illegitimate child in the putative father's will, incidental to an agreement to permit the adoption of the child by its father, where the adoption was in the best interests of the child and pecuniary gain was not the motivating factor on the mother's part.[48]

Another most important case on surrogacy in the USA was the decision in the Michigan case of *Doe* v. *Attorney General*[49] in which June and John Doe entered into a surrogacy arrangement with Mary Roe in terms of which she was to be artificially inseminated with John's semen, and bear a child which she would surrender to June and John on its birth. Mary was to be paid $5,000 and medical expenses. The Court of Appeals held that the adoption legislation did not prohibit surrogacy arrangements, but it did strike at payments. In Kentucky, the Attorney General challenged the activities of Surrogate Parenting Associates Incorporated who have a branch in the UK and were involved in the 'Baby Cotton' case. The Attorney General's argument was that surrogacy was prohibited by the statutes forbidding baby-selling. After a series of appeals, the Supreme Court held that the activities of the organization did not contravene the legislation.[50]

The most important case thus far is that of Baby M[51] a decision of the Superior Court of New Jersey. Mr and Mrs Stern were childless, because Mrs Stern suffered from multiple sclerosis and did not want to risk any debilitation which might result from pregnancy. Expert witnesses were of the opinion that this was a 'medically reasonable and understandable decision.' They had considered adoption, but their ages made adoption unlikely, but because Mr Stern, in particular, wished a child of his own, they employed a surrogate, Mary Beth Whitehead to bear a child for them, for which she was paid $10,000. She was artificially inseminated with semen from Mr Stern and bore a child, but because she refused to hand it over as she had agreed, the Sterns raised an action for custody. Mrs. Whitehead claimed custody as the natural mother. The efficacy of surrogacy arrangements were attacked on six grounds:

(i)   that the child would not be protected. The court stated that in the absence of legislation, it would protect the child;

(ii) that the surrogate would be exploited. The court was of the
      view that exploitation was more likely in private adoption
      rather than in surrogacy where the surrogate had an oppor-
      tunity before becoming pregnant of considering all the
      implications;
(iii) that to deal with a child for money denigrates human dignity.
      The court agreed, but was of the opinion that in a surrogacy
      arrangement, where the commissioning father is biologically
      related to the child, does not purchase the child;
(iv) that surrogacy infringes the adoption legislation. The court's
      view was the adoption legislation did not apply to surrogacy
      and that the only concepts which could apply were contractual
      ones and the principle that the child's best interests had to be
      considered;
(v)   that surrogacy will undermine the traditional concept of the
      family. The court asked 'How can that be when the childless
      husband and wife so very much want a child?'
(vi) that an elite upper economic group will use the lower group to
      'make babies'. The court regarded that argument as insensitive
      towards infertile couples.

The court considered that the contract should be fulfilled because
the surrogate was unsuitable to have custody and that the child's
best interests would be served by giving the Sterns custody.

Shortly after the decision in the case, it was announced that the
decision would be appealed and later, in the same year, the State
of Louisiana passed legislation prohibiting surrogacy.

However, although a surrogacy agreement might not infringe the
adoption legislation in respect of payment, the adoption provisions
have built-in safeguards for the child whereas these are not at
present imposed in relation to surrogacy.

In a state adoption there will be an investigation of the paternal
and maternal history of the child and also of the prospective adopters. Their financial position and motivation will also be considered.
Some or all of these factors may not be present in surrogacy. They
are present in adoption to ensure that what is done is in the best
interests of the child. However there are fewer controls over private
adoptions. In the USA some states prohibit these altogether,[52] but
in the remaining states and many other countries[53] including the
UK[54] they must still be in the best interests of the child. Private
adoptions are normally available only to relatives.[55]

Single persons employing a surrogate   These issues would arise in all
surrogacy arrangements. Where the person employing the surro-

gate is single a further problem might arise when he or she came to adopt the child. In some jurisdictions,[56] notably in the USA,[57] adoption by a single person is permitted only in exceptional circumstances, for example when it is not possible to find a suitable couple to adopt the child.

Employing a relative as a surrogate Some of the media coverage on this topic has been in respect of couples who have contemplated using a relative as a surrogate mother – usually the wife's sister.[58] In such a case, if payment or reward is not part of the arrangement, it would escape criticism on that ground. However the peculiar feature of such a practice is that the child's natural mother is still related to it, notwithstanding the adoption. In the usual adoption the legal and familial ties between the child and parent will be severed because the identity of the adopters will not be known to the natural parents, and vice versa. Where the surrogate is a relative however the familial ties remain. In some jurisdictions an adopted child may ascertain the identity of its natural parents and the child could find out that its natural mother is its aunt; the aunt will always have been aware of this. This special feature would have to be borne in mind and its possible effect on the child properly assessed. In March 1986 Steptoe and Edwards announced that they intended to use relatives as surrogates.[59] In South Africa in October 1987 a (grand)mother gave birth to a child for her daughter.

To conclude, a surrogacy arrangement would probably be unenforceable if it infringed either the letter or the spirit of the adoption or other legislation. If it does not, and there is no duress or some fundamental error about the nature of the agreement, it is difficult to see on what ground it would be thought objectionable and hence unenforceable.

Enforcement of the contract

If there is a valid contract a court may be asked to enforce it if either party fails to carry it out. That would be a breach of contract, and a court might order the defaulting party to implement the agreement. The breach might be so serious that it brought the contract to an end, or it might be of a lesser nature: in either case a claim for damages would be available, as it would if the party who was ordered to implement the contract nevertheless failed to do so. The agreement between the parties to a surrogacy arrangement might not be fulfilled for a variety of reasons.

For example, the surrogate might refuse to be artificially inseminated. That is a fundamental breach which would bring the contract to an end and the surrogate would have to hand back any money she had been paid. Damages would also be payable, but it is doubtful whether the intended nurturing parents would be compensated for any emotional loss which they might suffer, as the courts are reluctant to award damages under that head.[60]

Two other situations could give rise to a claim for breach of contract. The first is where the surrogate has an abortion. If an abortion was carried out because the child would be unlikely to live or would be severely defective, or where there was a threat to the mother's life, the courts would probably regard that breach as justifiable and make no award of damages, or award only nominal damages. If, however, the surrogate decided she did not want to continue with the pregnancy and had it aborted, a more substantial award of damages would be made, as her conduct would amount to an unjustifiable breach of contract and would also bring the contract to an end.

Where the surrogate conceives a child after embryo donation, it is as yet unclear which of the two mothers would be 'the mother' whose consent to the abortion would have to be obtained. One would assume that the carrying mother would be the appropriate person but the courts might consider the wishes of the genetic mother, especially if she is to be the nurturing mother. However it seems that the legislation has the carrying mother in mind and not the genetic mother.

Secondly a breach of contract might take place after the birth of the child. This could arise if the surrogate refused to hand over the child to the couple, or wanted it returned after she had given it to them, but before they had adopted it. The couple might be in breach if they refused to accept the child, or refused to keep it. In such circumstances two possible remedies would be open to the innocent party. One would be an award of damages, which in Anglo-American jurisdictions would be the primary remedy.[61] The other would be a court order requiring the other party to perform his side of the contract by handing over the child, which is called specific performance or implement.[62]

Where the surrogate mother refuses to hand over the child, the couple may have incurred expense, for example buying clothes for the baby, but if they have not suffered anything except perhaps emotional harm they might not be compensated,[63] except by nominal damages which would probably be regarded by them as unsatisfactory. As an alternative to the claim for breach of contract, the couple might have a claim in delict/tort for intentional or negligent infliction of mental or emotional distress.[64] Even if that was successful and a substantial award was made, the surrogate might not be able to pay.

The alternative to an award of damages is an order requiring the surrogate to hand over the child. Several points arise here. The first is that the courts are usually unwilling to involve themselves in contractual relationships of a personal nature. Thus they will not order one person to marry another where an engagement has been broken, nor will they force a person to join a partnership:[65] therefore they would probably not force a carrying mother to surrender her child, even if she was in breach of contract. That view is borne out by parts of the adoption legislation which permit a mother to change her mind until the adoption order is made.[66]

Another point about an order requiring performance of the contract is that it would decide who should have custody of the child. When that is in issue many jurisdictions emphasize the importance of doing what is in the best interests of the child.[67] An order requiring the surrogate to hand over the child could conflict with the 'best interests' principle. In the case of a very young child it will frequently be in its best interests to remain with its mother, but again the question may arise, which mother? However, if the surrogate was ordered to implement the contract, this would result in her being denied her parental rights in the child, and of course custody.

If the issue has to be determined according to the child's best interests, this will not be easy. Where the surrogate has been artificially inseminated by the male partner of the intended nurturing mother, the dispute would be between the natural mother and the natural father. The surrogate may have a strong psychological bond with the child, but the natural father would have a genetic link, and he and his partner would be prepared to create the same psychological bonds with the child. If the child was given to the natural father and his partner it would have two 'parents' and they might be better placed financially to provide for the child. Where the nurturing mother and her partner were also the genetic parents of the child, their claim would be even stronger.

Disputes between the surrogate and the intended nurturing mother and/or genetic mother would arise not only where the surrogate refused to hand over the child, but also where she wanted it back. There would be a similar dispute where the nurturing couple refused to take the child or refused to keep it.

The 'best interests' test requires a full consideration of the facts in each case. There will undoubtedly be cases where it might be thought to be in the best interests of the child to be with a party who, nevertheless, does not want it. Almost inevitably the child would be put up for adoption; but these 'tugs of love' are not a ground for objecting to surrogacy. Children are placed in similar unfortunate circumstances in many divorce actions.

There are a number of other ways in which the contract might be breached. The intended parents might wish the surrogate to refrain from smoking or taking drugs, to keep healthy and to attend antenatal clinics on a regular basis. If the surrogate did not do these things there might be a breach of contract, but it is doubtful whether it would be regarded as serious enough to permit the intended parents to regard the contract as at an end.

The problems of enforcement of the contract and remedies for any breach are therefore considerable. The courts may be unwilling or unable to award damages of the size which the party claiming them would wish. The difficulties faced by the courts are not peculiar to surrogacy and are not grounds for objecting to surrogacy agreements if they are enforceable.

In the only reported decision in the UK[68] a bachelor was living with a divorced woman who had had children, but could not have any more. They decided to pay a prostitute £3500 to have a child by being artificially inseminated by the man. One was found, and she accepted £3000. She was artificially inseminated and became pregnant. However, on the birth of the child she refused to hand it over, despite further inducements offered to her. The matter came before the courts, not on the issue of the enforceability of the contract, but rather on who should have care and control of the child and whether the couple, or more particularly the man, should have access. In the initial proceedings the child's mother was given care and control of the child and the father was granted access. The mother attempted to deny the father access and the issue came before the High Court. In the official report of the case the only matter dealt with is that of access. Comyn, J. gave the father access, but the Court of Appeal held the father should not have access.

It is clear from the newspaper reports that Comyn, J. made a number of observations on the arrangement between the couple and the prostitute. He described the agreement as 'pernicious' and hoped that the child, who was made a ward of court, would never be told 'the sordid story' of its birth. The issue of the enforceability of the agreement was not before the court, but it would not have been upheld. Whether the approach of Comyn, J. and the Court of Appeal was coloured by the fact that it was a prostitute whose services were hired is unclear, but again it seems likely that his comments were of wider application.

Even in the USA there have not been many reported decisions on surrogacy but the significant ones have already been discussed.

Status of the child

The question of how the child's birth ought to be registered has already been discussed, but the child's status is a different matter. A child may appear from the register of births to be legitimate, but this might not be the legal position. A child's status will conclusively determine to what extent it enjoys rights *vis-à-vis* its parents, whereas the entry in the register of births is not conclusive in that regard.

A legitimate child is entitled to full recognition as a member of its parents' family and enjoys certain rights as a result. The law determines who has that status and the rights which flow from it. In order to explain the status of the child born to a surrogate, it is necessary to say something about what the law regards as a legitimate child.

Legitimacy

At common law, in both Scotland and England, a child is legitimate if it is born or conceived at a time when its parents are validly married to each other; and there is a presumption that a child born during such a marriage is legitimate. The common law position has been altered to accommodate legitimation of a child by the subsequent marriage of its parents, and to make children of voidable, and certain void, marriages legitimate. Apart from these exceptions the position remains basically that of the common law.

In order to determine the status of a child born to a surrogate it is necessary to consider whether its parents were married to each other at the time of its conception or birth. If they were, it is their legitimate child and it is irrelevant that another couple are the intended nurturing parents. The relationships which can be brought within the term 'surrogacy' are set out in the Appendix, and while there are many permutations, the status of the children can be ascertained without too much difficulty. There are only two situations in which the child will be legitimate. The first is where a married couple decide to have their own child and hand it over to another person or couple after its birth. The child would be the first couple's legitimate child. The other situation is where a married couple's embryo is implanted into a surrogate. Again the child will be their legitimate child. In all other cases the child will be illegitimate. The child will therefore be illegitimate in the usual case of surrogacy where the surrogate is artificially inseminated by the male partner of the intended nurturing parents.

There is, however, a further complication where the surrogate herself is married. In this situation the child would be presumed to be the legitimate child of the surrogate and her husband. Usually the husband would not claim paternity, but he might if he and his wife decided to keep the child. The onus would be on the intended nurturing mother and her partner to prove, on the balance of probabilities, that the partner, and not the surrogate's husband, was the father. Where there is legislation on the status of the AID child, the surrogate's husband could be deemed to be the father and it might not be competent to prove the contrary.

Register of births

In addition to problems about status, surrogacy may also raise the issue who is the 'mother' of the child for purpose of registration of births. This would arise where the surrogate hosted an egg or an embryo. However, in respect of questions of status, it is the genetic or blood tie which is important, and not who actually gave birth to the child.

Conclusion

It would be foolish to suggest that surrogacy does not create legal problems and unrealistic to think that these can easily be overcome. Even if they could be resolved, there are other issues which would have to be considered. There is the ethical issue whether it is right for one woman to bear a child for another, and the social issue of the effect which such arrangements might have on the institution of marriage.

The arguments against surrogacy are many and convincing. In the past the relationship of marriage has been the principal way in which society produced children, and it was considered the most compelling reason for marrying. If surrogacy is to replace this, or be an alternative to it, a convincing argument can be put forward that it threatens the institution of marriage. On the other hand it may be that only a few people would be willing to employ this method, and that only a few would be prepared to act as surrogates. Moreover, even if surrogacy was regarded as acceptable for a couple, society might wish to prevent or dissuade single persons from using a surrogate. The arguments against this are that single persons are sometimes permitted to adopt children[69] and there is nothing to prevent a single woman having a child naturally or by artificial insemination.

One of the principal issues which has been discussed is the desirability of paying a surrogate. There are a number of commercial surrogacy agencies in the USA, and recently some of them have set up in the UK. The sums charged vary enormously, but commerical agencies are clearly in the business to make a profit. That could lead to exploitation of the surrogate, or the couple, or both.

It is probably unrealistic to expect a woman to become involved in a surrogacy arrangement without being compensated in some way, but the important question is whether surrogacy arrangements, if they are to be permitted, should be done on a commercial basis. There are good reasons why they should not be, and one is the possibility of exploitation, but possibly the main reason is the fear that women may agree to become surrogates only because of the money. There is clear and alarming evidence in relation to blood donation of the dangers which arise when blood donors are paid.[70] There is a temptation to conceal anything which might be prejudicial, and a surrogate might volunteer her services, for example, to finance her drug addiction. Furthermore the commercial element virtually dictates that only couples who can afford to pay will be able to use a surrogate. On the analogy of adoption, public policy would dictate that no payment be made, except for reasonable expenses. Other arguments are that commercial organizations may not achieve the standards which the medical profession apply in selecting donors and recipients in national AID programmes; and that the counselling which is offered in that connection may not be given to either the surrogate or the couple.

These are some of the arguments against commercial surrogacy, but if society disapproves of surrogacy in any form it is necessary to consider how the law might reflect society's attitude. One obvious approach would be to make it a crime for anyone to enter into a surrogacy agreement and for anyone to advertise surrogacy services, which has been done in the 1985 Act. (One agency whose activities have been referred to the Director of Public Prosecutions in England has attempted to get round the 1985 Act by paying the surrogates to keep diaries of their pregnancies.[71]) However it has recently been argued that this is 'too sweeping an approach'.[72] Several reasons are given for this. The first is that it might be difficult for the prosecuting authorities to prove that a surrogacy agreement had been entered into. If agreements are put in writing the problems would not be so great, but written agreements might be replaced by verbal agreements the existence of which would be more difficult to establish. The success of a prosecution might depend entirely on the parties admitting that they entered into the arrangement, and this seems unlikely.

Futhermore, as was pointed out in the *Lancet*[73] shortly after publication of the Warnock Report, a surrogacy agreement might be distinguishable from other legitimate activities only by the intentions of the parties. A couple might agree to donate semen, an egg or an embryo to a woman so that she could have a child. The only thing which would distinguish these donations from surrogacy is the intention that the child should be returned to the donor. Unless that intention was clearly recorded it might be impossible to prove. At present, for example, AID 'agreements' are not normally in writing, except in relation to consent.

Apart from the difficulty of proof, another issue which arises is whether society would wish to brand as criminals, infertile couples who wished to have a child and had explored all other possibilities and/or doctors who wished to help them, especially where there was no commercial element involved. (The Surrogacy Arrangements (Amendment) Bill 1985 sought to make all surrogacy arrangements illegal, whether they have a commercial element or not, but it failed.)

Society might wish to impose criminal sanctions only on those commercial organizations which practise for gain. Even these organizations would probably use verbal understandings rather than written contracts – having first been paid a substantial amount to ensure that whoever else lost out on the deal, they did not – or would disguise the true nature of the agreement.

The approach suggested by the Council for Science and Society is not to impose criminal sanctions, but rather to make these arrangements unenforceable in the civil courts. The parties could never ask the courts to enforce the agreement and surrogacy agreements would then be in a similar position to betting contracts. It would not be a criminal offence to enter into them, but the courts would not give their assistance if one of the parties wanted the agreement to be fulfilled by the other.

Having considered the arguments against surrogacy and how the law might deal with it, there is a case for permitting surrogacy provided adequate controls are imposed. Where a couple cannot have children they could be permitted to use the services of a surrogate, on certain conditions, for example:

(a) that there are medical grounds for saying that the woman cannot bear a child, or grounds for saying that she ought not to bear a child;
(b) that the practice must be medically supervised;
(c) that the surrogate bears a child after artificial insemination by the male partner of the 'infertile' woman;
(d) that each of the parties be adequately counselled, especially the surrogate. The surrogate would receive only reasonable expenses, which might include loss of earnings but would exclude any element of profit.

These conditions would go a long way to protect the parties from exploitation, and ensure that only surrogates who were genuinely interested in assisting those who could not have children would be used.

It is desirable that any arrangement be entered into formally, but that the agreement be kept as short as possible. In some of the commercial contracts there are clauses requiring the surrogate to attend ante-natal classes, refrain from smoking, and so on. While it is desirable that the surrogate should do these things it is imposs- ible to enforce such requirements, and if she does not carry them out the only remedy would be damages for breach of contract. A suitably motivated surrogate would probably comply with these conditions in any event. Another matter which cannot appropri- ately be dealt with in a contract is a change of mind by either party.

On balance, surrogacy may have a limited role; but never through a purely commercial or non-medical agency. As will be noted in the final chapter, the UK government does not intend to legislate further but surrogacy will be monitored by the proposed Statutory Licensing Authority.

PART IV
THE DOCTOR'S ROLE IN
ARTIFICIAL
REPRODUCTION

15 The doctor's role

In the preceding chapters it has been assumed that a doctor will be involved in the various processes which come under the heading of artificial reproduction.

In the majority of clinics in the UK a medically qualified person will be involved in the provision of AIH, AID, IVF and egg donation. In so far as surrogacy arrangements involve AID a doctor could be used, but some doctors may find this practice repugnant. The AID part of surrogacy would then be done by someone else and there has been some press coverage of instances where AID has been provided on a DIY basis.[1]

It is important to draw a distinction between AIH and AID on the one hand and IVF, embryo replacement and transfer and egg donation on the other. Both AIH and AID can be provided without involving a doctor. All the other processes require the skill of a doctor and probably of other professionals as well.

Because it is not necessary for a doctor to be involved in AIH and AID, his role has been described as 'more social than medical'.[2] That conclusion gives rise to social questions of considerable importance, for example whether society regards it as necessary or desirable to involve a doctor. If it is, should he act on his own or with others, and if so, with whom? Should the doctor have the final say in who are selected as donors and recipients of AID? If it is necessary or desirable to involve a doctor in AID, and legislation along the lines of that in the USA is contemplated, would the child be deemed legitimate only if a doctor had been involved?

At present, because a doctor is involved, the secrecy surrounding the identity of donor and recipients is virtually guaranteed. If others are involved who may not have any professional commitment to preserve secrecy, there may be a danger that greater publicity will be given to the service, which, in the past, has been regarded as undesirable.

The only legal issue arising is that any professional who is involved is required by law to exercise the skills of a reasonably competent member of his profession, and it cannot seriously be doubted that such involvement is reassuring to patients. If AIH and AID are provided by non-professionals, the recipients can have no such expectations.

The expectation of donors and recipients is that their identities will not be revealed; and the expectation of the recipients is that a professional person will display a certain standard of competence. These are sound reasons for involving a professional. The principal reason for involving a doctor is that the investigations of the male and female are recognized urological and gynaecological services, and genetic advice is given by the medical profession.

The selection of donors and recipients however has eugenic and social implications. It has recently been suggested that the counselling of couples prior to artificial reproduction should be carried out by trained personnel who are independent of the medical service to be provided. Research into artificial insemination has identified the need for this counselling service to be continuously available.[3]

Despite other uses which might be made of artificial reproduction techniques, their primary use will continue to be the alleviation of infertility. That being so, it is essential that medically-qualified personnel be involved. However, because the public has an interest in these activities, there should be some method by which that interest is represented.

One way is for local committees to oversee artificial reproductive techniques, with public representation on them. But that would not result in a consistency of approach from one area to another, and in any event they could be set up only under the authority of a statute. That being so, it would be preferable to have some national committee which would be responsible for overseeing these techniques throughout the UK, and any local committees – perhaps at Area Health Board level – would be answerable to the national committee. This point is taken up in Chapter 17.

PART V
THE WARNOCK REPORT
AND THE FUTURE

16 The Warnock Committee

In July 1982 the Secretary of State for Health and Social Services announced the setting up of a committee of inquiry into human fertilization and embryology.[1] The committee was chaired by Dame Mary Warnock, a distinguished philosopher at the University of Oxford, and it reported exactly two years later in July 1984.[2] Prior to Warnock there had been a number of discussions about artificial insemination,[3] but the Warnock Committee was the first to look at all of the new reproductive techniques, including artificial insemination, and their implications. Why it took until 1982 to set up such an inquiry is not clear, but the delay reflects on the various governments which have been in office since 1978.

By the 1970s AIH and AID were well established and the latter, at least, had been discussed frequently. By 1980 a number of children had been born as the result of IVF, and surrogacy was available in the UK and the USA. Furthermore it was known that scientists were researching on surplus embryos and there was talk of births from frozen embryos. The government is to be congratulated on setting up the inquiry and the Warnock Committee commended for producing its comprehensive Report so quickly. What still remains to be seen is the extent to which the recommendations of the committee will be implemented. It is suggested that it would be foolhardy not to follow the Report with legislative action. The present government has said that it will introduce proposals before the end of the 1988 parliament.

The committee's terms of reference were: 'To consider recent and potential developments in medicine and science related to human fertilisation and embryology; to consider what policies and safeguards should be applied, including consideration of the ethical and legal implications of these developments; and to make recommendations.'[4] They divided the task into two parts. First they examined the various procedures available to produce children for infertile couples. In the second part they looked at the benefits to be obtained by society from these procedures and related work.[5]

The distinction is not real, but is a convenient way of dealing with the subject.

The committee made several things clear at the outset.[6] They did not attempt to look at all the legal implications of the various practices they were considering. Instead they looked at the fundamental legal issues and confined their suggestions to essential legislative changes. However they cautioned against too speedy an intervention by the legislature in areas where the attitude of the public at large has not crystallized, but recognized also that both medical science and public opinion can alter 'with startling rapidity'.[7]

They looked at the techniques for overcoming infertility – artificial insemination, *in vitro* fertilization, egg donation, embryo donation and surrogacy.[8] Before dealing with the specific recommendations of the committee it is useful to note some general comments they make on the provision of infertility treatment.

General comments

They recommended that some services should be available under the NHS, and also in the private sector, to overcome infertility and hereditary disorders.[9] Each health authority should consider the infertility service which is currently provided and should consider establishing an infertility clinic which is separate from the existing gynaecological service.[10] The RCOG made a similar recommendation in 1982.[11] This would help to disabuse people of the notion that infertility is a gynaecological or urological problem and help to foster the idea that an infertile couple ought to be considered as a unit. The committee also suggested the establishment of a national group made up of central health departments to draw up guidelines on the organization of infertility services.[12] Other general principles included a recommendated that all infertile couples and donors ought to be given counselling both in the NHS and in the private sector.[13] Couples undergoing treatment should give full informed consent, and in the case of more specialized forms of treatment (which the committee did not list) consent in writing should be obtained.[14] I suggest that consent in writing ought to be obtained for all treatments dealt with by the committee, and that some thought ought to be given to the form of that consent: mention has already been made of the RCOG consent form for AID and this could be used as a model for other treatments.

Several important recommendations were made about donors. 'As a matter of good practice' they ought not to know the couple, and the couple ought not to know the donor.[15] However they did say that, while couples should not be able to choose donors on the basis of descriptions (by implication disapproving of semen banks containing, for example, semen from Nobel Prizewinners and the like), they ought to be given sufficient relevant information to reassure them. More important still, they recommended that at the age of eighteen the child should have access to 'basic information about the donor's ethnic origin and general health', and that legislation ought to provide for this. This is similar to the legislation on adopted children, but the important difference is that the child would not be able to identify his natural parent(s). While it may be important that a child should have this information at some point in his or her lifetime, it is suggested that the appropriate age is the age of marriage, namely sixteen, the time at which a person may first consider the implications of having a child. However there are good medical reasons why the child's general practitioner should be supplied with the relevant information at a very early stage, as it may be significant in treating the child. In their discussion on anonymity, the committee pointed out that 'on rare occasions a brother or sister' may be the most appropriate donor.[16] In such a case it is almost unavoidable that the child will know the identity of its natural parent; but whether or not these cases are numerous enough to allow such an exception, some further investigation is necessary into the social and psychological effects of using near relatives as donors. If it is desirable to use a relative, it is important that the child should not know of this at an early age.

The committee was also of the view that the NHS should keep a note of the number of donors and a separate list of the number of times each donor was used.[17] This would ensure that donors remained anonymous, but that the number of children produced from one donor should be known. They recommended that 'for the present' the maximum number should be ten, in order to avoid unwilling incest between children of the same donor. This limitation would apply to egg donors[18] and presumably also to embryo donors. There is undoubtedly a need for a limit, but views may obviously differ on the appropriate number.

They thought that semen donors should not receive payment, except for expenses.[19] This is in line with the practice in France[20] and the recommendation of the Council of Europe.[21] Their suggestion would apply also to egg donors and embryo donors. The principal reason for this recommendation has been mentioned earlier, namely that payment of a fee might tempt donors to conceal information which could result in their rejection.

One last general recommendation is that there ought to be a statutory licensing authority which would regulate infertility services and research, and this body would regulate who could offer infertility services and so on, and what they could do.[22] Shortly after the Report was published, the MRC set up its own monitoring body which has drawn up guidelines and inspected premises where infertility services are offered and research is carried out.[23] The research councils of other countries in Europe have also called for controls.[24]

There is at least one important matter which parliament would have to consider in connection with the proposed licensing body, and that is how the body would be constituted. The committee avoided detailed comment except to observe that the chairman should be a 'lay' person and that there should be substantial lay representation. It seems that 'lay' will be interpreted to cover professionals other than those in medicine and reproductive biology; because these practices raise legal, ethical and social issues and professional representation in those fields would be appropriate on the licensing body.

We turn now to the particular topics.

Artificial insemination by husband

The committee was of the opinion that this should continue to be offered, and made only one recommendation about AIH used during the husband's lifetime: that it should be administered by, or under the supervision of, a registered medical practitioner. [25] That would outlaw 'do-it-yourself' AI kits, which are available in this country and by importation; and they suggested that there ought to be legislative control over these kits which they thought should come within the ambit of the Medicines Act. However, as the licensing authority will be dealing with infertility services, perhaps it ought also to control them.

Artificial insemination by donor

The committee supported this practice and made an identical recommendation about its availability as that made in respect of AIH[26]

A very important recommendation, although it is not new, is that the AID child should be treated as the legitimate child of its mother and her husband where both have consented to the treatment.[27] This was suggested by the minority of the Feversham Committee,[28] and more recently by the Law Commission.[29] The Warnock Committee favoured a statutory presumption that the husband has consented, leaving it to him to dispute this if he so wished.[30] The reason, like that of the Law Commission, was that a child's status should not depend upon proof of consent or the existence of a document recording consent. Furthermore the legitimacy of the child would not be conditional upon the AID having been carried out by, or under the supervision of, a medical practitioner. Two other reforms follow from that. The first is that the donor's rights in and duties to the child would cease[31] and the second that the husband would be able to register himself as the father.[32]

While it is highly desirable that the child should be regarded for all purposes as the child of the husband or social father, it is suggested that some thought should be given to the question whether all the child's rights against the donor ought to be severed. The initial response might be yes; but there is a possibility, albeit remote, that the child would have a right to claim damages from the donor, for example because the donor deliberately concealed some material fact about his genetic make-up, and because this was not identified prior to birth the child was born handicapped. In such circumstances perhaps it is unjust to deny the child compensation, unless a no-fault scheme for compensating the child for any injury, no matter how it was caused is introduced. If the donor's rights are to be severed, it would be necessary to decide whether they ought to be severed from the time of donation, or from birth. Although it might seem odd to sever rights 'in the child' from the time of donation, given that there is no child and may never be one, it would avoid disputes between the donor and the 'parents' where the parties were known to each other. Section 27 of the Family Law Reform Act 1987 severs the link after birth. As already mentioned the committee recommended that on reaching the age of eighteen the child could obtain relevant information about the donor.[33]

Egg donation

This procedure is the corollary of AID. It requires some invasion of the donor's body to recover the egg, and at the time of the Report it had resulted in only one live birth.[34]

The committee favoured egg donation but subject to the licensing provisions already outlined.[35] They said however that this is one practice where a sister might be the only available donor, and noted that this would result in a breach of the principle of anonymity. For that reason they favoured counselling of all concerned, particularly about how and when to tell the child.[36] Legislation, similar to that suggested for the AID child, was recommended to deal with status, the rights of the donor and registration of birth.[37] The 1987 Act does not deal with this.

The issue raised in connection with AID of severing the child's rights against the donor and when that should happen also arises here. But in relation to egg donation – for example by a sister or other identified donor – there may be further complications. The donor might claim to be the mother of the child for the purpose of the Abortion Act and therefore try to prevent the carrying mother from having an abortion. As has been said, however, the Abortion Act gives rights only to the carrying mother.

In vitro fertilization

The committee looked at the arguments for and against IVF and recommended that it should continue to be available, subject to licensing;[38] that it should continue to be available on the NHS; and that the suggested working group should consider how an IVF service should best be organized within the NHS.[39] Its suggestions about surplus embryos are examined later.

Embryo donation

An egg which is fertilized *in vitro* may be implanted, not in the woman who produced the egg, but in another woman. The committee described this as 'embryo donation'. There are two different practices covered by this term. The first is *in vitro* fertilization of a donor egg with donor semen and the transfer or donation of the resulting embryo. This method was used in the first pregnancy from embryo donation.[40] The committee approved this method, and recommended that the child born as the result should be regarded in law as the child of the recipient couple, that they should register it as theirs and that the donors should not have any rights in the child.[41] This procedure, like AID and egg donation, would maintain the anonymity of the donor.[42]

The other method is to flush the embryo out of the donor's uterus, which is known as 'lavage', but there is a risk that the 'washing out' will not be successful and the donor will still be pregnant.[43] The committee concluded that this method should not be used at the moment in the UK.[44] In the first birth by egg donation, however, the donor was artificially inseminated and the embryo recovered by lavage;[45] so there seems to be a case for putting 'lavage' under the aegis of the licensing authority.

Surrogacy

The committee defined 'surrogacy' as previously described, namely an arrangement whereby one woman carries a child for another with the intention that it should be handed over after birth; and pointed out that it could take a number of forms.[46] They gave as examples of circumstances in which surrogacy could be used to alleviate infertility a woman who has no uterus or suffers from severe pelvic disease; other situations in which it might be used are where a woman does not wish to have a child because a pregnancy would interfere with her career.[47] It was noted that there is, at present, no provision in the NHS for surrogacy, and where it is undertaken it is usually through commercial agencies which charge a fee.[48] However, while surrogacy was not at the time illegal, the committee expressed the opinion that the courts would treat most, if not all, such arrangements as unenforceable.[49] That is clear by implication from the only UK case which has considered the matter[50] (and I and others have also expressed that view).[51]

The committee pointed out some of the practical and legal problems which can arise from such arrangements. For example, the commissioning mother might change her mind, she might die, or become disabled.[52] On the legal side, because a court would have to decide any dispute over the child on what was in the child's best interests, the committee thought it unlikely that a surrogate would be required to surrender a child if she did not wish to do so.[53] While one would accept this in a case where the surrogate is also the genetic mother, in situations where the commissioning mother is also the genetic mother, and where her husband is also the genetic father, the court might decide in her or their favour. Another point is that the father of the child could be liable to maintain it, no matter who was given custody of it.[54]

Having mentioned these factors, the committee looked at the arguments for and against surrogacy but unlike the other forms of treatment, they came out against surrogacy – by a majority – at least where it was undertaken by a commercial agency. Surrogacy has had a great deal of publicity since the publication of the Report. This point, previously mentioned in Chapter 14, is also dealt with in the final chapter.

Arguments for surrogacy

Having a child by a surrogate may be the only course open to a woman who cannot have a child of her own either because she does not produce eggs, or because she has some condition which prevents her conceiving. A woman who is advised against pregnancy would be in a similar position and her plight might be compounded if her husband was also infertile.[55]

The committee accepted that surrogacy could be seen as an act of generosity on the part of the surrogate and that there was no reason to suspect that surrogates would enter into such arrangements lightly.[56] The fact that a surrogate is paid does not, in itself, entail that there is exploitation either of her or the commissioning party.[57]

They also put forward counter-arguments to two other criticisms of surrogacy. The first is that it threatens the institution of marriage. A counter to that is that no one who is strongly opposed to surrogacy would become involved.[58]The point might also be made that it is unlikely that many people would opt for it even if it was the only course open to them. The small numbers of couples and women who would opt for surrogacy would hardly threaten the institution of marriage.

Secondly there is a bond between a mother and her child *in utero* which is broken by surrogacy. However, as the committee said, little is known about this bond, and even if it is important it is broken when the child is adopted.[59]

Arguments against surrogacy

The following arguments against surrogacy were mentioned by the committee: the bond between the mother and the child *in utero*; the undesirability of forcing a woman to surrender the child against her will; and that it is against human dignity for one woman to use her womb for profit.[60] These arguments persuaded a majority of the committee; but they admitted that, on that topic, they faced some of their most difficult problems.

All the committee agreed that surrogacy purely for convenience is ethically unacceptable,[61] but the majority felt strongly enough to recommend that it should be a criminal offence for agencies, whether profit-making or not, to operate within the UK, where the object is to recruit women for surrogacy, or couples who would avail themselves of surrogacy. The legislation should be sufficiently wide to render criminal the actions of those who knowingly assist in the establishment of a surrogate pregnancy.[62] Thus doctors and the commissioning parents would be criminally liable, although it is at least open to question whether a jury would convict in these circumstances. The Surrogacy Arrangements Act 1985 reflects some of the thinking of the committee.

Some observations on this approach and the arguments for permitting some forms surrogacy are discussed in Chapter 14; but this is one of the recommendations which has been met with some opposition. The *Lancet*[63] describing the committee's approach as displaying 'uncharacteristic ferocity' said that the implementation of their view would produce 'bad law inconsistent and unworkable', and felt that the continuing debate would reveal public sympathy for 'last resort' surrogacy. Similarly *Nature*[64] said that some surrogacy arrangements would be distinguishable from embryo donation only by the intention of the parties, which might not be disclosed; and suggested regulating surrogacy. These arguments repeat in essence the stance taken by the two members of the committee who dissented on this issue.[65]

In my view the law should have been left as it was at the time of the Report. Surrogacy agreements should not be criminal, but should not be enforced by the civil courts. Despite the passing of the 1985 Act, surrogacy requires a much fuller debate, not only on its commercial operation but also on the possibility of it being a part of infertility services. It was a mistake to legislate on commercial agencies until the implications for all other surrogacy arrangements had been thought out. A Private Member's Bill introduced in November 1985 sought to outlaw all surrogacy, but it failed.

Thus far we have considered the various techniques available to assist infertile couples to have children and the committee's conclusions. But there are other uses of these techniques and other issues such as freezing and research, which the committee also considered.

Transmission of hereditary disease and gender selection

There are circumstances in which AID is used, not to overcome infertility but to avoid the transmission of hereditary disease. Some of these diseases are transmitted by the male but, if his partner had AID, the child would not be affected. At present only AID has been used in this way, but if a hereditary disease, for example haemophilia, was transmitted by the female, egg donation would be appropriate, and in some cases where a hereditary disease might be passed on by either parent, embryo donation could be used. The alternatives for these people are abortion or the birth of children affected by these disorders. The committee thought that the use of donated sperm, eggs and embryos was acceptable in attempting to eliminate the transmission of these diseases.[66]

Allied to this are the techniques of selecting a gender for an embryo before fertilization and the identification of the gender of an embryo after fertilization. To have an embryo of a particular sex would clearly be beneficial to parents who run the risk of transmitting hereditary diseases. Although no successful method of selecting a child of a particular sex has yet evolved, it seems that this is not too far away. However as 'do it yourself' kits may be available the committee felt that these ought to be within the ambit of the Medicines Act.[67] If a method of 'sex selection' was available couples could use it for reasons other than the avoidance of hereditary diseases. The committee was unable to predict the likely effect of this, but recommended that the subject be kept under review by the licensing body.[68] Recently it has been announced that 'gender selection' has been practised at a Japanese university and this has caused great controversy.[69]

Freezing and storage

The use of frozen human semen was developed in the early 1950s and is now commonplace. However, a safe and reliable method of freezing human eggs has only recently been developed. Children have been born from embryos which have been frozen, and in July 1986 the first birth from an egg which had been frozen was reported.

The advantages of freezing semen, eggs and embryos are that the persons who produced them do not have to be available for their subsequent use. Furthermore where embryos are frozen they can be reimplanted in a woman should an earlier attempt at implantation fail. This would avoid having to recover her eggs and fertilize them *in vitro* before each implantation.

The committee recommended the continuing use of frozen semen, but suggested that a child conceived by AIH which was not *in utero* at the date of death of its father should be disregarded for the purposes of succession to his estate.[70] The committee specifically mentioned succession rights and so a child conceived in this way would not, even under their proposal, forfeit rights of maintenance from the estate. This recommendation is somewhat strange, because it puts the posthumously-conceived child in a worse position than an illegitimate child. Secondly a posthumously-conceived child may be conceived not long after the death and would be almost indistinguishable from a child conceived immediately prior to death, but not born until after it. Lastly very few people would want to produce a large number of children in this way. It was suggested earlier that a child conceived in this way should have succession rights in the husband's estate but that there should be a limited period within which a child conceived by this method would have such rights.

Even if the committee did not wish to encourage posthumous conception, their recommendation does not take account of a case where a woman was inseminated at a time when, it was later established, her husband was dead. An example would be where a husband died in a road accident or at work at say 9 a.m., by which time his wife had left to go the clinic where she was inseminated at 9.30, still unaware of his death. On the committee's recommendation, the child would be illegitimate and denied succession rights since it could be shown conclusively that the woman was not inseminated until after her husband's death. A similar difficulty arises within their proposal on IVF.

It is suggested that this difficulty could be overcome by providing that any child born by AIH or AID shall be illegitimate and disregarded for the purposes of succession to and inheritance from the husband unless the insemination occurred during his lifetime or at any time when his wife was unaware of his death. A similar proposal would cover IVF but instead of 'insemination' one would have 'replacement or placement of the embryo in the woman'.

On the use of human eggs the committee felt that frozen eggs should not be used for therapeutic purposes until it was clear that no unacceptable risk is involved, and recommended that the matter ought to be reviewed by the licensing body.[71] They also recommended that the clinical use of frozen embryos should continue, again subject to review.[72]

The committee discussed the ownership of semen, eggs and embryos after the death of the depositors. The problem is particularly acute with embryos. If these are items of property which can be bequeathed by one couple to another, a child subsequently born would have four parents. To avoid this and other problems the committee sensibly recommended that where a person dies during the storage period the right of disposal should pass to the storage authority.[73] They also suggested a periodic (five-year) review of stored semen and eggs,[74] and recommended that embryos should be stored for a maximum of ten years after which the storage authority should have the right of disposal.[75] A period 'of the order of ten years' was also recommended by the National Health and Medical Research Council of Australia,[76] but a much shorter period of one year was recommended by the BMA. The reasons given by Warnock for a definite time limit were: 'current ignorance of the possible effects of long storage . . . and the legal and ethical complications that might arise over disposal of embryos whose parents have died or divorced or otherwise been separated'.[77] With all due respect to the committee, this reasoning is unsound since the problems can arise no matter how short the storage period is. The committee made separate recommendations dealing with the death of both parents and situations in which they cannot agree about use or disposal of the embryos.[78] The only valid argument is that based on the long-term effects of storage, but within the ten-year period the couple have the right of use or disposal, and so there does not seem to be any good reason why they should not have the right also to determine the period for which the embryo would be stored.

A slightly different proposal had to be made about embryos where one of the partners died. The committee suggested that in that event the right to use the embryo should pass to the survivor.[79] Where both died (the committee did not add 'or could not be traced') the right should pass to the storage authority.[80] This eminently sensible suggestion would circumvent the problem which arose in Australia where a couple who had an embryo which was frozen subsequently died in a plane crash. The question arose whether the embryo should succeed to their estates or be implanted in another woman or be allowed to die. The balance of views seemed to be that the embryo had no right to succeed, but the Attorney-General for Victoria decided that the embryo should remain frozen until the state had clarified the issues.[81]

If the couple could not agree on the use or disposal of the embryo, the committee recommended that the right should pass to the storage authority.[82] This recommendation requires further thought. It should be obvious that couples may agree on a matter one day and disagree the next, but the committee's view would not permit a change of mind by the couple. It is therefore suggested that the right to determine the use of the embryo should pass to the storage authority only after the expiry of the ten-year period. Although the phrase 'use or disposal'[83] looks like the concept of ownership, the committee recommended legislation to ensure that the sale of human gametes or embryos should be permitted only under licence from the licensing body.[84] This may avoid some problems, but it still leaves the possibility that a couple or the storage authority could donate an embryo to close relatives within the ten-year period. Given that there are prohibitions against marrying within particular degrees of relationship, it would be necessary to have legislation to prevent this.

The committee also made recommendations about succession rights of children conceived from embryos which have been frozen. They were of the view that for this purpose the important date should be birth and not the date of fertilization.[85] The firstborn would therefore be the eldest for succession purposes where being the firstborn is significant, as it would be in relation to titles of honour. Also on the issue of succession, the committee made a suggestion about posthumously conceived children, similar to that mentioned in connection with AIH.[86] The comments made there are equally applicable here.

Research on human embryos

This is an area of considerable complexity on which there are widely-differing views, and in the Report itself there are two dissents.[87] This issue prompted considerable comment in the press immediately after publication of the Report;[88] and it will continue to be discussed. The crucial issues facing the committee were whether research on human embryos should be allowed and, if so, in what circumstances and subject to what controls. They did not define the term 'research' but said that it covered two broad categories of activity. The first – pure research – is aimed at increasing knowledge of the human embryo in its early stages. The second – applied research – has direct relevance for patients who are infertile in that it assists with diagnosis or treatment. They excluded new and untried treatment undertaken in an attempt to alleviate infertility.[89]

For many, no doubt, research on human embryos means (or perhaps conjures up images of) experimenting with them or manipulating them in some way to see how they react, but it is important to note that research may mean no more than using a microscope to observe the various stages of development of the embryo.[90] If someone says he is opposed to research on human embryos, it would be necessary to find out exactly what he means by 'research'. This is particularly significant in relation to the committee's recommendation that 'no embryo which has been used for research should be transferred to a woman'.[91] It would be essential to have some definition of 'research' even if it only said what was excluded from the definition.

Arguments against research

Some people are fundamentally opposed to research on human embryos and their stance is a moral one. For them, the embryo is a human being, or a potential human being, and entitled to the same protection as other humans. Research can take place on humans only with their consent, and because embryos are incapable of giving consent research cannot be carried out. Furthermore any research might deprive the embryo of its life or potential life.[92] Others feel that research is tampering with human life and express fears about 'mad scientists' or 'mad governments' producing anomalous creatures or indulging their theories on breeding and eugenics.[93]

Many who are opposed to research accept that a great deal of valuable information may be lost, as may opportunities to detect, limit or prevent inherited disease, but they regard the moral principle as taking precedence.[94]

Some of these arguments, raised by three members of the committee in Expression of Dissent B, refer to the majority view that research could be carried out until the fourteenth day after fertilization, but accepted that thereafter the moral principles and the law would afford the same protection to the embryo as they do to other humans. However the three dissenters made this comment: 'Before that point has been reached the embryo has a special status because of its potential for development to a stage at which everyone would accord it the status of a human person. It is in our view wrong to create something with the potential for becoming a human person and then deliberately destroy it.'[95] The dissenters supported the creation of embryos with a view to 'their ultimate implantation in the uterus' and suggested that any embryos remaining after implantation should 'either be frozen with a view to implantation at a later date or allowed to die'.[96] This raises at least two points of controversy. One is that many would not accept the argument that the embryo is morally distinguishable from sperm and egg, nor the premise based on potential.[97] Furthermore it is by no means generally accepted that there is a valid moral distinction between deliberately destroying an embryo and allowing it to die.[98] However, despite these observations, there are many who would undoubtedly share the sentiments expressed in this Dissent.

Arguments for research on human embryos

The committee clearly had widely-differing views put to them on this also. Some thought that respect (or protection) must be afforded only to persons, and did not regard human embryos as persons, or even potential persons. That was a view held by a minority. The more commonly expressed view was that human embryos are entitled to more respect than animal subjects, but that the respect or protection cannot be absolute and must be measured against the benefits to be had from research.[99] It might be suggested that this leaves the moral position and, perhaps also, the legal position in some doubt, if protection is not absolute. However, in a carefully-researched article Professor Gordon Dunstan traced the history of the protection afforded to embryos and noted that it varied with the stage of development. He also observed that the notion that protection is given from fertilization can be traced to the mid-nineteenth century and no earlier.[100] Even if the moral position of the embryo is in doubt, as the committee noted there is no doubt that in law the human embryo has no status and no right to life. The committee referred to abortion and damages for injury *in utero* and noted that neither supports the argument that the human embryo *in vitro* has any protection.[101]

In the committee's view, however, the human embryo should be given some protection. Their recommendation was that research should be allowed to continue, but only under licence, and that the unauthorized use of an *in vitro* embryo should constitute a criminal offence. The committee observed in a footnote (although it is an important matter and directly related to their discussions) that their proposal to regulate work on human embryos in their early stages would look odd if there was nothing regulating the use of foetuses and foetal material for research.[102] This was the subject of inquiry in 1972, but the Report concluded that, while there was nothing which prohibited research, equally there was nothing which permitted it either.[103] The Warnock Committee suggested that urgent consideration be given to this matter.[104]

Another important recommendation was that research on human embryos should not continue before fourteen days after fertilization.[105] That date is the one suggested by the BMA, the MRC, the Royal College of Physicians[106] and the Ethics Advisory Board (EAB) in the USA.[107] (One thing which is worth noting is that the committee's recommendation related only to 'any embryo resulting from *in vitro* fertilisation' and would not restrict the type or duration of research carried out on embryos resulting from *in vivo* fertilization. That would require to be clarified in legislation.)

The period of fourteen days after fertilization corresponds with the time at which implantation would take place and also the appearance of the 'primitive streak' which is the first of several identifiable features of the development of the embryo.[108] However, 'the evidence showed a wide range of opinions on this question'[109] and other time limits have been suggested. In their evidence to the committee, The Royal Society felt that the time of implantation was too restrictive since it did not take into account 'the important question of embryonic organisation'.[110] It did not however suggest a specific alternative. The RCOG concluded that the appropriate cut-off point was day 17, being the point when early neural development begins.[111] At one time Steptoe and Edwards wished to develop embryos to day 30, which is when the brain begins to develop. This would allow more extensive research into genetic diseases, and one of the arguments in favour of this is that brain death marks the end of life; brain development could therefore be said to mark its beginning.[112]

Given the differing views there is an argument for having a period fixed, not by legislation, but by the licensing authority, or by the Secretary of State. It may be that further research in this area will prove, as the Royal Society suggests, that fixing a limit at day 14 is unduly restrictive. It would be easier for this to be changed by the Secretary of State after consultation than it would be to alter legislation.

Another matter which was an integral part of the committee's discussion was the recommendation that consent should be obtained from the couple not only for research on spare embryos but also for the method of use or disposal.[113]

Hitherto the committee had discussed the use of spare embryos, but they recognized that embryos can be created solely for research and are not always a by-product of *in vitro* fertilization. Four members were opposed to the deliberate creation of embryos for research.[114] To allow this, they argued, would be inconsistent with the special status that the committee as a whole wished to confer on the human embryo. They were also concerned that the deliberate creation of embryos in this way might open the door to 'less valid research'.[115]

Other members did not share that view. Their stance was that if research was to be permitted on human embryos, it was irrelevant why the embryos were created.[116] This seems the correct approach. The committee recommended a special status for the human embryo and it would acquire that no matter how or why it was created. The majority therefore favoured research on these embryos, but subject to exactly the same controls as those for 'spare' embryos.[117]

Future developments

The committee went on to consider possible future developments,[118] given that some public anxiety had been expressed.[119] The specific future developments examined were trans-species fertilization, the testing of drugs on human embryos, ectogenesis, gestation of human embryos in other species, parthenogenesis, cloning, embryonic biopsy, nucleus substitution and the prevention of genetic defects.[120]

Prevention of genetic defects[121]

What the committee was considering here is related to the earlier discussion about overcoming genetic disorders. As previously noted, they approved the use of AID, egg donation and embryo donation to achieve this end.[122] It may become possible to identify genetic defects at an early stage in the embryo's development, and one or more of the embryo's genes could be replaced to remedy the defect. Public anxiety has been expressed not on the therapeutic use of such a technique, but in respect of its possible use to produce human beings with specific (and presumably 'desirable') character-istics, that is, selective breeding or 'eugenics' in the pejorative sense. The committee suggested that the licensing body should draw up guidelines as to what types of research would be considered unethical and would not therefore be licensed. These guidelines would be reviewed periodically to take account of scientific advances and changes.

Trans-species fertilization[123]

Some trans-species fertilization is currently practised in the investigation of male infertility. It has been ascertained that apparently sterile men whose sperm will fertilize a specially treated hamster egg may be able to father their own child, rather than have to resort to AID or adoption.[124] The eggs fertilized in this way will not develop beyond the 2 cell stage.

The committee noted that it might be possible to use other species and the public have expressed concern about the development of hybrids – the modern centaurs. They regarded trans-species fertilization as acceptable when it is part of a programme for diagnosing or alleviating infertility or sub-fertility, but they saw no reason why such creations should be allowed to survive beyond the 2 cell stage. They recommended that anyone who developed a hybrid beyond that stage should be guilty of a criminal offence and that trans-species fertilization should be done only under licence.[125]

Testing drugs on human embryos.

It was pointed out to the committee that newly-developed drugs and other preparations might be tried out on human embryos to see whether they were toxic or likely to cause abnormalities. They realized that this might concern people because embryos might be 'mass-produced' for this purpose, and they were of the view that this was not acceptable because a large number of embryos would be required. They did not close the door entirely, however, recognizing that there may be exceptional circumstances which would justify such tests 'on a very small scale'. This would also be a matter for the licensing authority.

This may give the licensing authority some cause for concern. A pharmaceutical company might be able to put forward a convincing case for using embryos to test drugs for use during pregnancy. Before the drugs would be accepted a large number of trials would have to be done and the issue facing the licensing authority would be whether this should be permitted. The pharmaceutical company might very well be sued if it had not carried out a sufficient number of trials; but if the appropriate number of trials were permitted on embryos it would be difficult to argue that this would still be 'on a very small scale'.

Ectogenesis[127]

Ectogenesis means developing an embryo in an artificial environment, with the ultimate aim of producing a child by this method. The arguments in favour are that it would enable studies to be undertaken of normal embryos and foetuses and would permit some women to have children who would otherwise have to use a surrogate. The committee saw no reason to depart from their recommendation that embryos should not be sustained for longer than fourteen days. This development is well in the future and it may be that similar information can be obtained by other means. It is, of course, a notion central to Aldous Huxley's *Brave New World*.

The usual objection to procedures like ectogenesis is that they ought not to be permitted until the likely effects are known. It is none the less clear that these will not be ascertained until ectogenesis is tried. It may be possible however to assess ectogenesis by the study of premature babies. At present babies of about twenty-four weeks' gestation can survive, and by gradually improving techniques to save babies of even shorter gestational age more information can be gathered about the likely effects of a child born by ectogenesis.

Gestation of human embryos in other species[128]

Some animal embryos have been gestated in the wombs of other species. For example, the wombs of rabbits have been used to carry cow embryos.[129] However the relevant animal work does not suggest that this would be possible in humans. The committee recognized that someone might attempt this and therefore suggested that it be a criminal offence. Presumably the committee's view was that there were no identifiable advantages in such a practice.

Parthenogenesis[130]

This term is applied to a reproductive process whereby a gamete, usually an egg, develops into one of the species without fertilization – resulting in so-called 'virgin birth'. The committee's information was that such a development would not take place in the foreseeable future – despite a recent book in which it is suggested not only that it is possible, but that it has happened[131] – and they made no recommendation or other comment on it. In view of the claims made in the book, however, this is another matter which ought to be kept under review by the licensing body.

Cloning[132]

There are two types of cloning one of which was identified by the committee, that is, where the 2 cell embryo is divided into two separate cells. At this point each cell can continue to grow and the result would be identical twins. This merely mimics what occurs naturally. This process has been successful in animals, notably frogs,[133] but the committee said that, to the best of its knowledge, it had not been done successfully in humans. However it could be developed in humans to produce a genetically-identical clone. The clones would be the same age, unless one was frozen and later thawed. Dr Edwards has suggested that this type of cloning could assist with research into inherited defects. One embryo could be examined to see its gene structure, and if it was defective it would not be implanted.[134] Given the close link with other work on early embryos, it is submitted that this type of cloning ought also to be within the remit of the licensing authority. The committee did not, however, make any recommendation about cloning of this kind.

The other type of cloning raises even more fundamental issues. This involves removing a cell from an *adult* and allowing it to develop. At the 2 cell stage the embryo cells have not differentiated into blood cells, nerve cells and so on, but thereafter they do, and so in order to make a clone from an adult's cell, the cell would have to be treated in some way so that it loses its specialist character. It is generally thought that this cannot be done despite a claim by David Rorvik in 1978.[135] Rorvik tells the story of 'Max' who hated leaving anything to chance. For that reason he had never had any children. Max was a man of ability and had a strong constitution. He wanted to be sure of passing his qualities on to a child and this cannot be guaranteed with normal reproduction. Accordingly, Rorvik claimed, a scientist removed a cell from Max and eventually produced an identical genetic clone. This is probably a fiction, but several distinguished scientists have taken the possibility seriously,[136] and Rorvik puts forward a plausible reason why an adult would wish to have a clone. The reason is similar to that behind the organization of the 'Nobel prizewinners' sperm bank in California which was set up in 1980. (The first child conceived with semen from this bank was born in April 1982, and is called Doron.)

The central issue is whether a society would wish to be able to mass-produce clones, thus reducing, but not eliminating, human differences. This may not be undesirable on a limited scale, but would have to be controlled. Unlike the first type of cloning, the second is probably not of immediate significance and therefore there would be no justification for keeping it under review until it seemed possible.

Embryonic biopsy[137]

This would involve removing some cells from the embryo in order to investigate its chromosomal structure. The embryo would not be damaged and would be frozen until the cells had developed and been examined. If they did not reveal any abnormality, the embryo would be thawed and implanted. The committee found it difficult to estimate how likely it is that embryonic biopsy will be developed in the near future. One disadvantage they mentioned is that it involves IVF. They went on to say: 'Given the present relatively low success rates for pregnancy following IVF, it is unlikely that embryonic biopsy will become a feasible method of detecting abnormal embryos for some considerable time.'[138] This reasoning is hard to follow. Embryonic biopsy is carried out on embryos, admittedly with the intention of implanting them if they are not abnormal, but its feasibility does not seem to be related to the success rates for IVF. In any event one of the pioneers of IVF, Dr Robert Edwards, has suggested that IVF might eventually achieve a higher success rate than natural reproduction, for two reasons: first that IVF verifies that fertilization has taken place; and secondly that it is possible to discover whether or not the embryo seems to be developing properly. He forecast a success rate of one pregnancy for every two embryos implanted.[139]

As it may be possible to work on embryonic biopsy during the period of fourteen days suggested by the committee, this seems to be another topic for consideration by the licensing authority.

Nucleus substitution[140]

The technique sometimes referred to as cloning means the removal of the nucleus from a fertilized egg and, without hindering its subsequent development, replacing it with a nucleus from an adult. Edwards has suggested that this might be used to replace defective organs in adults.[141] The committee made no recommendation on nucleus substitution, but it is quite clear that work on animals is going on in this area, and again it would be appropriate to refer it to the licensing authority.

In making its recommendations on these topics the committee had to balance two distinct sets of interests, both clearly identifiable and both perfectly legitimate. The first is the duty of the scientist (be he doctor, physiologist or whatever) to inquire into the order of things and by so doing further our knowledge of human reproduction, genetic diseases and so on. The other is the need to reflect public opinion on these issues, and work within an accepted ethical framework.

Throughout the Report the committee mentioned views which have been put to them, but felt that they had not been contacted by as many people as might have given information.[142] They also frequently mentioned public concern and were of the opinion, rightly, it is submitted, that the public interest might be reflected somehow in these areas:[143] 'A society which had no inhibiting limits, especially in the areas with which we have been concerned, questions of birth and death, of the setting up of families, and the valuing of human life, would be a society without moral scruples. *And this nobody wants.*'[144]

The committee believed that all the techniques they had described, (with the exception presumably of those about which they made no recommendation) required 'active regulation and monitoring, even though, as we realise, such restrictions may be regarded by some as infringing clinical or academic freedom'.[145] But, as they rightly said, all 'doctors and scientists work within the moral and legal framework determined by society'.[146] However, they said that they did not wish to interfere with the capacity and freedom of the doctor to exercise clinical judgment. The committee's object was that these activities should be placed 'on a properly organised basis within a framework broadly acceptable to society'.[147]

To achieve this, they recommended a new statutory licensing authority to regulate both infertility services and research.[148] They did not make particular comment on the size of the body nor on its composition, but as it would be required to assess medical and scientific work there would clearly have to be a significant representation of these disciplines. But they did recommend that there should be substantial lay representation and a lay chairman.[149] It is somewhat surprising that there was constant reference throughout the Report to the ethical and legal implications of these techniques, but that no suggestion was made that either a lawyer or a moral philosopher, or both, ought also to be on this body. It is clear also that infertility and research work has sociological implications and the licensing authority would have to be made aware of them. The licensing authority could, however, be given power to co-opt members for certain limited purposes.

The particular topics to be referred to the licensing authority have been mentioned, but the committee also considered the general functions of this body: it would issue general guidance on good practice in the provision of infertility services and on the types of research which are acceptable; it would offer advice to the government and be available for consultation; and so that the public could be made aware of what was happening, it would publish an annual report. These are the advisory functions.[150] It would also have an executive function to cover the granting of licences to those offering infertility services and to researchers.[151] The specific provisions relating to licences have already been mentioned.

While it is for parliament to decide what powers the licensing body should have, it is suggested that it should appoint officials with power to inspect premises to ensure that they are licensed and that only work permitted under the licence is being carried out.[152] It is suggested also that the person in charge of the premises covered by the licence should prepare and submit annual reports to the licensing authority, and other reports if requested.

The committee's recommendation that a licensing authority should be set up was 'by far the most urgent', and without the creation of such a body none of their other conclusions could have any practical impact.

There can be little doubt that the committee was faced with an enormously difficult task – not only because of the large number of different topics within their remit, but also because of the complex issues surrounding them. To be able therefore to report comprehensively in two years is a remarkable feat.

17 The aftermath of Warnock

As was to be expected, the publication of the Warnock Report in July 1984 resulted in an enormous amount of media coverage. Much of the initial reaction was favourable,[1] but within a very short time the Report was criticized, substantially on two fronts – surrogacy and research on human embryos. Indeed these two issues have continued to occupy most of the post-Warnock discussion, almost to the exclusion of other topics.[2] For example there has been little public discussion about the provision of infertility services and one could easily conclude that the public cares very little about them. That may not be so, but surrogacy and research on human embryos have undoubtedly been the topics most widely discussed. In this chapter we shall look at some of the more important developments in the United Kingdom and also in other countries since the Report was published.

Immediately on publication the Department of Health and Social Security and the Scottish Home and Health Department invited comments on the Report by 31 December 1984 in order to assist the formulation of the government's response.[3] It was expected that the government would thereafter announce when it intended to introduce legislation, and expectation was heightened first by a court case on surrogacy, and secondly by the introduction by Enoch Powell of a bill – the Unborn Children (Protection) Bill – to restrict research on human embryos. However, during the Second Reading of the Bill all that the Health Minister, Kenneth Clarke, would say was that legislation would be introduced as soon as was feasible.[4] That remains the position in December 1987 and although parliament has not seen the proposed legislation, both Houses debated the Warnock Report: the House of Lords on 31 October 1984[5] and the House of Commons on 23 November 1984.[6] In November 1987, a White Paper was published revealing a possible framework for legislation[7] and it is also to be debated in both Houses.

The debate in the House of Lords

This debate lasted over four hours and almost thirty peers took part. Most of the speakers concentrated on research on human embryos and surrogacy and in relation to surrogacy it was accepted that commercial arrangements should be outlawed, and private ones discouraged.[8]

In the discussion of research on embryos, many were opposed to any kind of research without indicating what they actually meant by that term.[9] Some used the term 'experiments' and would not allow experimentation on human embryos.[10] Not surprisingly there were calls for a temporary or permanent moratorium on 'research' and/or 'experiments'.[11] Among those unsympathetic to the Warnock recommendations on research, a number made statements about life beginning at fertilization or conception or that a unique human being resulted from fertilization.[12] It is somewhat unfortunate that these speakers did not draw a distinction between fertilization and conception, and that they made these statements despite the evidence that there can be no certainty until the fourteenth day after fertilization that there will be only one embryo. For example, Lord Denning could say: 'I have read the scientific evidence, and from the moment of fertilization . . . there is a different new being – a living being.'[13] That comment was made immediately after the speech by the Bishop of Chelmsford who had said: 'The argument for the 14 day limit is that individuation is not complete until 14 days. I am told that up to that point, for example, the embryo may split and form twins.'[14]

Almost inevitably in such a debate, there were a few speakers whose comments demonstrated an almost irrational fear of progress in these areas. Lord Rawlinson of Ewell talked of surplus embryos in this way: 'They are potential living things, human rats or rabbits, the creation of "spares" but alive . . . If society permits some of its members to treat human life in accordance with the proposals of this Report, we move inexorably down a path which will lead to a monstrous society, ultimately of fabricated creatures.'[15] Viscount Buckmaster ended his comments on experimentation with the cautionary words, 'So, apart from all the horrible results of experimentation, we may even have hermaphrodites with us.'[16] These comments were all made by speakers who were either wholly opposed to the findings of the Report or at least opposed to research on human embryos.

By contrast, there were two well-balanced and well argued speeches from Lord Soper[17] and Lord Prys-Davies[18] and a good summing up by Lord Glenarthur.[19]

Lord Soper's comments were mainly directed to research on

human embryos and surrogacy. In dealing with research, his view was that whatever the potential of the embryo, any harm which might be done to it had to be balanced against the benefits to be gained from the modern methods of reproduction. He also made a most pertinent observation:

> I am not particularly impressed by the arguments that one must not indulge in any research on any one of the spare embryos which necessarily will be produced in this way. It is clear to me that there is no greater moral value in saying that we must just allow the spare embryo to die, or to say that we can indeed make use of them for future culture or for future ways of delivering them ourselves from these particular difficult and complex problems.[20]

On the issue of surrogacy, he found himself 'in the greatest of difficulties'. He went on to say that if there was 'the slightest taint of commercialism' he would be opposed to it, but he did not rule out surrogacy in all circumstances.[21]

Lord Prys-Davies thought that the Warnock Committee had 'maintained the right balance' on the issue of research and on surrogacy.[22] He shared the views of the two dissenters on the Warnock Committee on the subject of surrogacy,[23] as did Lady Masham.[24] Lord Prys-Davies raised a very important issue which was outwith the remit of the Warnock Committee, namely the question of what priority was to be given to IVF and other forms of treatment in the National Health Service. The problem of the allocation of NHS resources is a subject of continual discussion but is almost insoluble.

Taken as a whole the speeches in the House of Lords, with a few notable exceptions, did not explore the issues in as much depth as the Warnock Committee and there were, regrettably, a number of speakers who stated their views almost as dogma, in the teeth of the scientific evidence. Few displayed any knowledge of the subject and many were willing to impose a moratorium, as Lord Glenarthur said in his summing-up, without thinking about what would happen after it had been removed.[25]

The debate in the House of Commons

The debate which took place in the House of Commons less than a month later was no more enlightening. It opened with a statement by the Secretary of State for Social Services,[26] who almost congratulated himself for having the foresight to appoint the Warnock Committee in 1982. According to him, the public debate over the implications of the first 'test tube' baby in 1978 had not developed to anything like the condition it had in 1984. While that may be true, many of the implications could have been discussed profitably in 1978. They were discussed by Dr Edwards on many occasions, for example in his important article in 1974;[27] and by 1978 surrogacy had received some press coverage.[28]

A number of MPs stated that the embryo was unique, or was entitled to protection from the time of fertilization or conception, but again no clear distinction was made between these and there was little reference to the scientific evidence.[29] Most of the speakers were opposed to research on human embryos and also to surrogacy, but there was little discussion of what was meant by the term 'research' or what types of surrogacy should be banned. However there were some balanced and thoughtful comments, notably from Michael Meacher[30] and Leo Abse[31] but also, as in the House of Lords debate, some less well-balanced and thoughtful outbursts.[32]

The debate was summed up for the government by Kenneth Clarke, the Minister for Health. He admitted to having modified his views and indicated that it was difficult for him to arrive at certainty on some of the issues. He did however make the following important comment: 'What is needed here is a set of laws and rules which the right minded majority of society will accept, given that we approach the problems with tolerance of the range of views and life styles in a country such as our own.'[33]

The developments since the debates have been mainly in surrogacy and research on human embryos.

Surrogacy

This is the only topic on which there has been legislation since the publication of the Report. The reason for this was a controversial case of surrogacy which came before the High Court in England in January 1985.

As noted in Chapter 16, the Warnock Report advocated that surrogacy should be banned. It was therefore somewhat ironic that the day following its publication it was announced that four surrogates had signed contracts agreeing to carry children for other women in exchange for £6500. The contracts had been entered into with an American organization, the National Centre for Surrogate Parenting, which has been operating in the United Kingdom since 1983.[34] Following that announcement, although not necessarily as a result, there was further press comment. Most of it appeared to be opposed to surrogacy but no clear distinction was drawn between cases (a) in which there was a commercial agency involved and those where there was not; (b) or in which there was a financial consideration and others where there was not. Shortly thereafter the *Lancet*[35] and *Nature*[36] published comments from scientists who were of the opinion that in some circumstances surrogacy ought to be permitted, but that couples might have to accept that the agreement they entered into would not be legally enforceable. In August 1984 *The Times* carried an item about an Australian surrogate who refused to hand over the child to the commissioning couple,[37] which is what had happened in an English case in 1978.[38] Early in 1986 there was a similar case in New Jersey.[39]

After August 1984 little more was said until January 1985 when it was disclosed that a child had been born to one of the four surrogates, Mrs Cotton (who has written her own account of the whole matter).[40] She was willing to hand over the child but the local authority, who seemed in some confusion over the whole issue, obtained a 'place of safety order' for the child under the Children and Young Persons Act 1969. Most lawyers regarded this step as inappropriate or incompetent, because the Act is designed to deal with children who are neglected by their parents or who are likely to be ill-treated by them or whose health is likely to suffer as a result of being with their parents.[41] It was not intended to deal with children born to surrogate mothers. However before the matter could come before the Juvenile Court the child was made a ward of the High Court by, it was thought, the natural (commissioning) father. On 8 January Mr Justice Latey imposed a ban on publicity and gave his judgment on Friday, 11 January: it was not delivered in open court until Monday, 14 January, by which time the child had left the jurisdiction. The judge decided the case on the child's best interests, and concluded that the natural father should be given custody and gave him leave to take the child abroad.[42] There is little doubt that the decision was sound, and it was shrewd to give it on the Friday and allow the couple time to leave the country anonymously before his judgment came under scrutiny. The judge was obviously satisfied that the commissioning couple were willing to have the child and provide a suitable home for it. The circumstances surrounding its conception and birth were, in his view, irrelevant. The sole issue was the best interests of the child.

The day before the decision was announced, the Health Minister said that the government would decide soon about how to deal with commercial surrogacy;[43] and very shortly thereafter the Surrogacy Arrangements Bill was introduced. It became the law on 16 July 1985. The Act, in brief, bans commercial surrogacy agencies and surrogacy carried on by or through such agencies.[44] It does not however penalize either the surrogate or the doctor, but that would have been the result if the Surrogacy Arrangements (Amendment) Bill, introduced into the House of Lords on 28 November 1985, had

become law. It did not, and in the recent White Paper the government has disclosed that it does not intend to legislate further on
surrogacy, but it will be kept under review.[45]

Parliament has therefore taken the approach suggested by
Warnock, of making some surrogacy activities criminal, rather than
simply rendering the arrangements unenforceable. This approach
has also been adopted in Germany.[46] Despite the ban however
surrogacy continues. One organization, Reproductive Freedom
International, has attempted to circumvent the legislation by paying
surrogates, not for carrying the children but (as previously
mentioned) for keeping diaries of their pregnancies. Their activities
were being considered by the Director of Public Prosecutions in
England but nothing seems to have resulted.[47] On 8 March 1986
Steptoe and Edwards announced that they would use relatives as
surrogates and that they would be unpaid.[48] Mr Steptoe later called
for legislation to clarify the position of children born to surrogate
mothers.[49]

There is undoubtedly some support for surrogacy in limited
circumstances but it is clear that it should be the subject of careful
control, as the British Medical Association said at its Annual
Representative Meeting in June 1985.[50] This is the sensible
approach, rather than imposing a total ban which was the aim of
the Surrogacy Arrangements (Amendment) Bill. It may be cynical
to say so, but surrogacy will continue, even on a commercial basis,
no matter what legislation might say. It is surely better to have
the activity controlled and medically supervised than carried out
clandestinely and without proper medical back-up. These factors,
as we shall see, have persuaded the Law Reform Commission of
Ontario to propose control of surrogacy in Canada. Surrogacy
would however be permitted provided that it is medically indicated
and the whole arrangement is supervised by the court.

The other two recent developments on surrogacy, viz the English
case which considered the issue whether a surrogacy arrangement
which included a payment infringed the Adoption Act and the
Baby M case in New Jersey have been discussed in Chapter 14.

Research on human embryos

The other major topic which has attracted attention is research on
human embryos. Central to the discussion is whether they are
human beings and entitled to full protection, or not human beings
and hence entitled only to limited, or no protection. As one would
expect there is a wide spectrum of opinion and most of the publicity
has been given to those who are opposed to all research on human

embryos. It was announced in parliament on 15 February 1985 that
two million people had signed a petition against research on human
embryos.[51]

Without going into too much detail (most of which can be gleaned
from the Warnock Report) the two views most commonly adopted
can be seen, on the one hand, in a letter to *The Times*[52] from
Professor M. C. Macnaughton, President of the Royal College of
Obstetricians and Gynaecologists, who favours research; and on
the other in the Unborn Children (Protection) Bills, the first of
which was published on 18 January 1985, whose sponsor Enoch
Powell is against research. Although Powell's bill was defeated
other Unborn Children (Protection) Bill were introduced in the
House of Commons on 21 October 1985, 4 December 1985, 10
December 1986 and 28 October 1987. None, except the Powell Bill
got a Second Reading, and the Powell Bill did not get beyond that.

In his letter to *The Times* Professor Macnaughton said that experiments on human embryos may assist in the prevention of
conditions such as Down's Syndrome, cystic fibrosis and muscular
dystrophy. In addition information about the growth of embryos
may help to prevent or reduce miscarriages and the birth of babies
with abnormalities. He argued that the advantages of the research
should be weighed against the disadvantages of not being able to
eliminate these and other disorders.

The object of the Unborn Children (Protection) Bills was to ensure
that the approval of the Secretary of State was obtained for the
following activities, viz: (i) the fertilization of human eggs *in vitro*;
and (ii) the possession of the resulting embryo. Only married
women could seek *in vitro* fertilization under the proposed legislation and the embryo could be used only for implantation, defective or not. This proposal, if it had become law, would have reduced
the provision of *in vitro* fertilization, if not removed it, and it would
certainly have outlawed all research on human embryos. No scientist would be irresponsible enough to implant a defective embryo
into a woman: yet that is what the legislation would have required.
A defective embryo, even if not implanted, could not have been
studied in order to ascertain why it was defective. The Bills failed
to become law, but the Powell Bill, in particular, had a great deal
of support. Many would, undoubtedly, have been unaware of the
precise implications of the proposed legislation, for, at the very
least, the titles of the Bills using the word 'children' were grossly
misleading, possibly deliberately so.

However, while the Powell Bill was in Parliament, the MRC and
the RCOG announced the setting up of a Voluntary Licensing
Authority[53] perhaps to allay the fears of those who supported the
Powell Bill. The Authority has produced two Reports,[54] but it will

probably be replaced by the Statutory Licensing Authority envisaged by Warnock and now more of a reality since the publication of the most recent White Paper.[55]

Despite the hope of many that the government would legislate soon after the publication of Warnock, as has been noted earlier in this chapter, these hopes faded. Even with the publication in June 1986 of a White Paper,[56] it was clear from the title that it was yet another consultative paper and by no means clear that legislation would follow soon, if at all. Hopes have however, been raised by the most recent White Paper which, as it says, is a framework for legislation, but even that will be debated in both Houses of Parliament and on the one major issue, viz: research on human embryos, the government has not expressed any view and it will be left to a free vote in Parliament.[57] The government will adopt the somewhat unusual tactic of having a Bill with alternative clauses. Given the poor quality of the previous debates, the prospects for informed debates on the recent White Paper and the Bill are not high.

Some things are however, clear. The government proposes a Statutory Licensing Authority (SLA) which will license individuals, establishments and activities, including research on embryos, if that is approved.[58] There will be criminal sanctions for any breaches of the licensing provisions.[59] Even if research is permitted, some activities will be forbidden. These include the creation of hybrids, cloning and trans-species fertilization.[60] There will be detailed provisions dealing with the control and storage of embryos,[61] but it interesting to note that the government does not propose to forbid the use of semen or embryos after the death of their 'creators'.[62]

As has been noted, the position on surrogacy is that it will be monitored by the SLA, but no further legislation is envisaged. The existing Act will remain and will not therefore be extended to all forms of surrogacy.[63]

Two other major matters are covered in the White Paper and they deal with the children who are born as the result of the gamete and embryo donation. The bizarre situation where children in England and Wales (but not in Scotland) who are born as the result of AID are deemed to be the children of the consenting husband[64] will be remedied by having legislation for Scotland and the legislation will be extended to cover egg and embryo donation.[65] Warnock favoured giving these children access to some information about their natural parents on the model of adopted children,[66] but the government recognizes that there are differences and so does not make any recommendation.[67]

Despite the indications that legislation is at least proposed, it remains to be seen when a Bill will be introduced and what its fate will be, particularly on research on human embryos. It would seem that the other topics will be enshrined in legislation with little or no opposition.

The UK government has been slow to act in the field and that can be contrasted with the position in other parts of the world, notably Australia, and to a lesser extent in the USA, Canada and Europe.

Canada

There is, as yet, no legislation in Canada on *in vitro* fertilization, but various bodies, for example in British Columbia,[68] Alberta[69] and Saskatchewan[70] have discussed artificial insemination. However, there is legislation only in Quebec and Yukon.[71]

In 1985, the Ontario Law Commission produced a comprehensive Report covering most of the issues discussed by the Warnock Committee in the UK.[72] The Report contains recommendations on artificial insemination, *in vitro* fertilization, research on human embryos and surrogacy. Among other things it recommended the regulation of artificial insemination,[73] and that the consenting husband should be deemed to be the father of the child.[74] On *in vitro* fertilization, the Report has recommendations on storage, control and disposal of embryos,[75] and in relation to research, it approves a 14-day cut-off point, as had been suggested by Warnock.[76] On surrogacy it suggested legislation to regulate the practice, and it is interesting to note that, far from wishing to ban it, it recommended that the surrogacy arrangement should be supervised by the courts.[77]

USA

As noted in chapter 8, a large number of states have legislation on AID., but in the mid–1970s, the Department of Health Education and Welfare (DHEW) imposed a moratorium on IVF. However in 1979 the Ethics Advisory Board of the DHEW consider the legal and ethical issues arising from IVF and its advice was that IVF was ethically acceptable, and furthermore that it ought to be given federal support. It recommended that a model code be drafted which would contain provisions about the status of children conceived as a result of IVF and the rights of the parents, doctors and others involved.[78] As yet no draft has appeared. However in Illinois, Pennsylvania and New Mexico there is legislation on IVF. The Illinois statute provides that a person who fertilizes an egg *in vitro* becomes its custodian for the purposes of an 1877 Act on Child Abuse.[79] Although this might seem to expose the doctor to possible liability, in a case which was decided after the Act, it was held that the doctor would contravene the legislation only if he wilfully injured or endangered the embryo either by abusing it or carrying harmful experiments on it.[80] The Pennsylvania Legislation creates a regulatory framework for IVF by requiring that certain information be publically recorded, for example the names of the parties involved in the clinical processes, the number of eggs fertilized, the number of those subsequently discarded, and the number of women who have had eggs re-implanted.[81] The statute in New Mexico is one of many which restrict experimentation on foetuses and embryos but it is the only one which mentions IVF in that context.[82] There have been several cases on surrogacy and there is one statutory provision. These have been mentioned in Chapter 14.

Australia

Thousands of children have been born in Australia as the result of AID and more than a thousand as the result of IVF.

The Australian Law Ministers first discussed the legal status of children born as a result of AID in 1977, but following the birth of Candice Reed in 1979 the Ministers called for an urgent report on the legal issues which arise from IVF and other new reproductive techniques. In 1980 it was decided that uniform legislation on the status of children born as a result of AID should be enacted in all the Australian jurisdictions. The legislation would provide that the husband who consents to his wife undergoing AID should be deemed to be the father of any child born as a result, and that the sperm donor should have no rights or liabilities in respect of the child and *vice versa*.[83]

As a result of the test-tube births in Australia, all six State Governments and several other bodies established Committees when enquiry to consider *in vitro* fertilization and in some cases also the practice of AID. Between 1982 and 1987, each one of the State Governments received at least one Report on the new birth techniques.[84] As yet, the New South Wales Law Reform Commission has still to complete its enquiry which began in 1983. These Reports have recommended that there should be legislation to regulate these new birth techniques.

Victoria In Victoria the IVF Committee has produced three Reports, one on donor gametes, one on the disposal of embryos and one on surrogacy.[85] These Reports were produced between 1982 and 1984. Much of the discussion in Victoria arose out of the death of Mr and Mrs Rios in a plane crash. Their embryos had been frozen and a decision had to be reached on how to deal with them.

The Victoria Law Reform Commission recommended in August 1984[86] that the embryos should be destroyed, but almost immediately the legislature ordered that this should not be done.[87]

In May 1984, the Victorian Government passed the Status of Children (Amendment) Act which came into force on 1 August, the same date as similar legislation in New South Wales. The Act creates a presumption that the husband is the father of the child and it deals also with the status of children born after egg donation or embryo donation. In such cases there is an irrebuttable presumption that the woman who gives birth to the child is the child's mother and this is coupled with an irrebuttable presumption that the egg donor is not the mother. In addition, in November 1984 the Infertility (Medical Procedures) Act was passed. That Act was based almost entirely on the recommendations of the Victorian IVF Committee. The Act provides that IVF procedures may be performed only in approved hospitals and for married couples who have previously had treatment for infertility which has proved unsuccessful. It also deals with record keeping and the provision of information about donors to the Department of Health. It provides for the setting up of a body which would review IVF and advise the minister on this and also on other measures used in connection with the alleviation of infertility. This body is also the body which would consider research projects.[88]

The IVF Committee had earlier recommended that there should be a prohibition on the sale of human gametes and this also appears in the Infertility (Medical Procedure) Act. The Act does, however, permit a gamete donor to be paid for both travelling and medical expenses.

In the third report the IVF Committee considered surrogacy. The Committee concluded that commercial surrogacy should be prohibited because it was of the opinion that the essence of a surrogacy arrangement was the buying and selling of a baby. The 1984 Act prohibits advertisements and the offering of surrogacy services and also the giving or receiving of any awards or payments for such services. The Act also provides that surrogacy contracts are void and hence unenforceable. The Act deals however with commercial surrogacy only and therefore it does not affect other kinds.

New South Wales The Law Reform Commission of New South Wales produced a discussion paper on human artificial insemination in 1984 and a Report in 1986.[89] The Report has 42 recommendations on the broad areas of the regulation of artificial insemination, the donor (including recruitments, selection and screening, eligibility for AID, counselling and consent, unanimity, confidentiality, storing of semen, posthumous artificial insemination, record keeping and the legal liability of the participants. As yet no legislation has followed but in 1984 the Artificial Conception Act was passed. It came into force on 1 August 1984 and provides that, where a husband consents to AID he is irrebuttably presumed for all purposes to be the father. The husband's consent is presumed but that is a rebuttable presumption. There is another irrebuttable presumption that the donor is not the father. The Act provides that the terms 'husband' and 'wife' include partners of the opposite sex where the parties are living together on a *bona fide* domestic basis.

In July 1987 the Commission produced a discussion paper on *in vitro* fertilization.[90] It concluded that there are many aspects of IVF which do not call for special regulation, provided that the practice is confined to the medical profession. It was of the opinion that IVF and associated research can be accomplished without blanket licencing requirements, and without restricting the practice to particular kinds of institutions.

It was of the opinion that eligibility for IVF should be a matter to be determined by medical experts but it tentatively proposed the creation of a State Advisory Committee with a multi-disciplinary membership to oversee the whole area.

It proposed that there should be legislation providing that a woman who bears a child by means of artificial conception who intends to raise the child should conclusively be presumed to be the child's mother. Where a child was born as a result of the use of stored reproductive tissues, the paper concludes that it would be reasonable for the law to provide that the stored conceptus should not be regarded as the child of the testator for the purposes of inheritance unless specific provision is made about it in the testator's will. The legislation would also provide that the clinic has power to determine the use, storage and disposal of reproductive tissues donated to it.

On research the Commission did not think there was any persuasive reason to restrict or prohibit research on human embryos entirely. It thought that the community would favour such research provided that there were time limits laid down and provided that there were reasonable constraints and that the persons carrying out the research should be accountable, supervised and forced to keep records. The Report also deals with record keeping, consent, counselling and legal liability.

In May 1987 the Commission produced a research report on surrogate motherhood which was the result of a national sample survey of Australian public opinion.[91]

The results were that a total of 51 per cent were not opposed to surrogate motherhood and there was clear support for providing some form of payment to the surrogate. Eighty-three per cent favoured the payment of medical expenses and some 40 per cent found the payment of an agreed fee acceptable.

The majority view was that the parties themselves should be free to make the necessary arrangements but there was majority support for the existence of non-profit making agencies.

The issue which was most controversial was that of the enforcement of the arrangements. The opinion poll revealed that approximately a third were of the view that in the event of a dispute the married couple should have the first claim to the child. Approximately 26 per cent would favour the surrogate mother in such circumstances, whereas another 25 per cent thought that the courts should decide. It is interesting to note that approximately 80 per cent of those consulted did not approve of surrogacy for other than medical reasons.

South Australia   A Working Party on IVF and artificial insemination reported in January 1984[92] and following on that the Family Relations Amendment Act 1984 was passed which adopted the scheme of the Victorian Legislation.

Queensland   In 1984 a Special Committee reported on artificial insemination, *in vitro* fertilization and other related matters. Like the Warnock report it was comprehensive in that it dealt with the ethical, social, economic and political issues as well as the legal ones.[93] It is understood that Queensland is in the process of considering legislation on these topics.

Tasmania, Western Australia, Australian Capital Territory and The Northern Territory   All these jurisdictions have legislation on the status of children following the pattern of the Victorian legislation.[94]

One other development which is worth noting is that in April 1985, a private member introduced a Bill into the Federal Parliament, the aim of which was to prohibit much of the research on human embryos. As a result a Senate Select Committee was set up to consider this Bill and it produced a Report in September 1986.[95]

The Committee first addressed itself to the important question of what is an 'embryo' and what is meant by 'experimentation'. The Warnock Committee did not attempt to define the term 'embryo' but the Select Committee thought it should be used to describe the post-fertilization and further stages up to the point where the human form emerges. The Committee thought that, in connection with experimentation, a distinction should be drawn between therapeutic and non-therapeutic experimentation, but it recognized that it would be impossible to reflect a unanimous view and it is not surprising therefore that 2 out of the 7 members dissented on this aspect.

In the Committee's view, the embryo was not an item of property, but it was an entity which should be protected by having a guardian. Accordingly, it had to be protected against destructive non-therapeutic experimentation.

The Committee thought it desirable that the whole of Australia should recognize uniform ethical standards in relation to embryo experiments and it is recommended the setting up of a national body to evolve a research protocol and to be responsible for policing the licencing procedures for institutions and personnel. In its view, these proposals should be enshrined in a Commonwealth statute which would impose criminal sanctions for infringement. As yet no further action has been taken.

Europe

The Council of Europe produced its draft report on Human Artificial Insemination in 1979 but more recently, in November 1985, its Committee of Experts on Medical Research on Human Beings met in Strasbourg to consider the principles upon which human artificial reproduction should be regulated. A draft was considered at another Meeting in Trieste in July 1986 and a final draft was prepared in April 1987 for submission to the Committee of Ministers in December 1987.[96] The draft deals with the storage of gametes and embryos and states the need to fix a maximum period for preservation. It is recommended that posthumous use of the semen of a deceased husband or partner should be prohibited.

The Report reiterates the earlier thinking that donors of eggs, sperm and embryos should not be paid, but that the cost of collection, removal, conservation and implantation of gametes or embryos may be recovered.

The final draft suggests that maternity should be determined by the fact of giving birth rather than genetic origin and that as far as paternity is concerned a husband who has consented to artificial procreation would have no right to contest paternity. It goes on to suggest that in order to promote the integration of the child into the family all legal obligations and relationships between the child and the gamete or embryo donors should be severed, provided the donation is made through an authorized establishment.

The last important subject which was covered is that of surrogacy. The general view was that surrogacy should be prohibited. The final draft however does say that states may, allow surrogacy in exceptional circumstances provided that there is no material gain.

Elsewhere

Although there have been considerable developments in the United Kingdom, Europe and Australia, and to a lesser extent in some respects in the USA and Canada, there is little evidence of activity elsewhere in the world. It is not surprising that such developments as there are have taken place in the areas just mentioned. Despite these developments and the careful consideration given to the implications of the various issues arising from the new reproductive techniques, it is interesting to observe that in March 1987 the Vatican declared that *in vitro* fertilization is morally unacceptable.[97] This opinion will not, of course, have gone unheeded but it will be interesting to see whether mention is made of it in either of the two debates in the United Kingdom on the Government's legislative proposals.

Conclusion

It is to be hoped that the United Kingdom Government will produce legislation along the lines which it has indicated and given the various developments, particularly in Australia, it is highly desirable that a Statutory Licencing Authority be set up with powers to monitor the new reproductive techniques. In the writer's opinion, it would be unfortunate if the SLA did not also have the power to regulate human embryo experimentation. It is quite clear from a survey carried out by the Times in October 1982 and a Marplan Poll conducted in 1985[98] that a majority of people in the United Kingdom are in favour of some form of experimentation on human embryos, presumably because of the benefits which they perceive from such work. It will be interesting to see whether, in a year from now, the position in the United Kingdom is any different.

Appendix: Artificial reproduction

	Sperm	Egg	Gestational mother	Intended parent(s)
1	*Artificial insemination by husband*			
	Mr A	Mrs A	Mrs A	Mr & Mrs A
2	*Artificial insemination by partner*			
	Mr A1	B1	B1	Mr A1 & B1
3	*Artificial insemination by donor*			
	Mr A1	Mrs B	Mrs B	Mr & Mrs B
	Mr A1	B1	B1	B1 (& partner 1,2)
4	*Confused artificial insemination*			
	Mr A1 & Mr B1	Mrs A	Mrs A	Mr & Mrs A
	Mr A1 & Mr B1	Mrs C	Mrs C	Mr & Mrs C
	Mr A & Mr B1	C1	C1	Mr A & C
	Mr A1 & Mr B1	C1	C1	C1 (& partner 1,2)
5	*Egg donation (ovum donation)*			
	Mr A	B1	Mrs A	Mr & Mrs A
	Mr A1	B1	C1	Mr A1 & C1
6	*In vitro fertilisation and embryo replacement*			
	Mr A	Mrs A	Mrs A	Mr & Mrs A
	Mr A1	B1	B1	Mr A1 & B1
	Mr A1	B1	B1	B1 (& partner 1,2)
7	*Embryo donation*			
	Mr A	Mrs A	Mrs B	Mr & Mrs B
	Mr A	Mrs A	B1	B1 (& partner 1,2)
	Mr A1	C1	Mrs B	Mr & Mrs B
	Mr A1	C1	B1	B1 (& partner 1,2)

	Sperm	Egg	Gestational mother	Intended parent(s)
8	*Surrogate motherhood*			
	Mr A	Mrs A	B1	Mr & Mrs A
	Mr A	B1	B1	Mr & Mrs A
	Mr A	B1	C1	Mr & Mrs A
	Mr A1	B1	B1	Mr A1 (& partner 1,2)
	Mr A	B1	C1	Mr A1 (& partner 1,2)
	Mr A	Mrs B	Mrs A	Mr & Mrs B
	Mr A	Mrs B	C1	Mr & Mrs B
	Mr A	B1	Mrs A	B1 (& partner 1,2)
	Mr A	B1	C1	B1 (& partner 1,2)
	Mr A	Mrs A	Mrs A	Mr & Mrs B
	Mr A	Mrs A	Mrs A	B1 (& partner 1,2)
	Mr A	B1	Mrs A	Mr & Mrs C
	Mr A	B1	Mrs A	C1 (& partner 1,2)
	Mr A	Mrs A	B1	Mr & Mrs C
	Mr A	Mrs A	B1	C1 (& partner 1,2)
	Mr A	B1	C1	Mr & Mrs D
	Mr A	B1	C1	D1 (& partner 1,2)
	Mr A	B1	B1	Mr & Mrs C
	Mr A	B1	B1	C1 (& partner 1,2)

Notes
1 = married or unmarried
2 = male or female

Notes

Chapter 2

1. Behrman, S. J. and Kistner, R. W. 'A rational approach to the evaluation of infertility' in Behrman and Kistner, p. 1, Newill, R., *Infertile Marriage* (Harmondsworth, Penguin, 1974), p. 13.
2. In 1984 (the last year for which statistics are available) there were 395 800 marriages in the UK, *Population Trends* no. 44. London, HMSO, 1986. In 1982 there were 2 495 000 marriages in the USA. This figure is provisional but is the most recent available, *Statistical Abstracts of the United States of America 1985*. United States Department of Commerce, Bureau of the Census.
3. Behrman and Kistner, p. 4; Newton, J. R., 'Current status of AI in clinical practice', in RCOG (AI), pp. 25–41; Saunders, D. M., 'The assessment of the infertile couple for AID' in Wood, pp. 38–49; Guttmacher, A. F., 'The role of artificial insemination in the treatment of human sterility', *Bull. NY Acad. Science* (1943), 119, pp. 573–91, at 589; Verkauf, B. S., 'Artificial insemination: progress, polemics and confusion – an appraisal of current medico-legal status', *Houston LR* (1966), 3, pp. 277–309, at 283.
4. Stangel, J. J., *Fertility and Conception: an essential guide for childless couples* (London, Paddington Press, 1979), ch. 4; Harrison, R. G. and de Boer, C. H., *Sex and Infertility* (London, Academic Press, 1977), ch. 3; Philipp, E., *Childlessness: its causes and what to do about them*. London, Arrow, 1975; IPPF, *Handbook on Infertility*. London, 1979; Consumers' Association, *Infertility*. London, 1969.
5. Harrison and de Boer, op. cit., p. 28; Guttmacher, A. F., op. cit., at 581. Others use a lower figure, eg. 20m/ml, see Dixon, R. E. and Buttram, V. C., 'Artificial insemination using donor semen: a review of 171 cases', *Fert. and Ster.* (1976), 27, pp. 130–4, at 130, or 10–15m/ml.; see Behrman, S. J., 'Artificial insemination' in Behrman and Kistner, p. 779.
6. Chester, R., 'Is there a relationship between childlessness and marriage breakdown?', *J. Biosocial Science* (1971), 4, pp. 443–54.
7. (England & Wales) Bromley; Cretney; (Scotland) Clive; (USA) Krause, *Family Law*.
8. Adoption (Scotland) Act 1978 s. 13; Adoption Act 1976 s. 13.
9. Adoption (Scotland) Act 1978 s. 15; Adoption Act 1976 s. 15.

Chapter 3

1. Epstein, I., ed., *The Babylonian Talmud*. London, Soncino Press, 1938.
2. Hag. 14b–15a.
3. Lev. 21:13 (AV).
4. Rosner, F., *Studies in Torah Judaism: modern medicine and Jewish Law* (New

York, Yeshiva University, 1972), p. 91; Kardiman, S., 'Artificial insemination in the Talmud', *Harofe Haivri: Hebrew Medical Journal* (1950), 2, pp. 164ff.

5. Ginzberg, L., *The Legends of the Jews* (Philadelphia, Jewish Publication Society of America, 1968), VI, 400–1.
6. Schellen, A. M. C. M., *Artificial Insemination in the Human* (Amsterdam, Elsevier, 1957), pp. 8–9.
7. ibid. p. 288.
8. ibid. p. 9; Rohleder, H., *Test-Tube Babies: a history of the artificial impregnation of human beings* (New York, Panurge Press, 1934), p. 35; Finegold, W. J., *Artificial Insemination*, 2nd edn. (Springfield, Ill., Thomas, 1976), p. 5.
9. Schellen, op. cit., p. 10.
10. ibid.
11. ibid., p. 11.
12. ibid., p. 13.
13. ibid., p. 13.
14. Home, E., 'An account of the dissection of an hermaphrodite dog' in *Phil. Trans. Royal Society*, vol. 18, pp. 157–78, at 161–2; Schellen, op. cit. p. 13.
15. Schellen, op. cit., p. 18.
16. Hard, A. D., 'Artificial impregnation', *Medical World* (1909), 27, pp. 163–5.
17. McIntosh, T. M. in ibid., p. 196; Hamilton, N., ibid., p. 253; Newth, C. H., ibid., p. 197; Egbert, C. L., ibid., p. 253; Barton, E., ibid., p. 305.
18. Newth, op. cit.
19. Barton, op. cit.
20. Hard, op. cit., p. 306.
21. Schellen, op. cit., p. 20; Behrman, S. J., 'Artificial insemination' in Behrman and Kistner, pp. 779–89, at 779; Klugman, S. J. and Kaufman, S. A., *Infertility in Women* (Philadelphia, Davis, 1966), p. 168.
22. Seashore, R. T., 'Artificial impregnation', *Minn. Med.* (1933), 21, pp. 641–3.
23. Seymour, F. I. and Koerner, A., 'Artificial insemination, present status in the USA as shown by a recent survey', JAMA (1941), 116, pp. 2747–9.
24. Folsome, C. E., 'The status of artificial insemination: a critical review', *Am. J. Obs. & Gyn.* (1943), 45, pp. 915–27; Guttmacher, A. F., op. cit., pp. 577–9.
25. Feversham Report, App. 1, 'The law and practice overseas: United States of America', pp. 91–2.
26. Curie-Cohen, M. *et al.*, 'Current practice of artificial insemination by donor in the United States', *NEJM* (1979), 300, pp. 585–9.
27. Barton, M., Walker, K. and Wiesner, B. P., 'Artificial insemination', *BMJ* (1945), 1, pp. 40–3.
28. Feversham Report, paras 21–3.
29. BMA Panel, pp. 3–5.
30. Report by the RCOG. The author is grateful to the College for permission to refer to this survey.
31. Feversham Report, App. 1, 'The law and practice overseas', para. 4.
32. Hahlo, H. R., 'Some legal aspects of human artificial insemination', SALJ, 74, pp. 67–174, at 169.
33. Leeton, J. F., 'The development and demand for AID in Australia' in Wood, p. 10.
34. Hill, A. M., 'Experiences with artificial insemination', *Aust. & NZ J. Obs. & Gyn.* (1970), 10, pp. 112–14.
35. ibid., p. 10.
36. ibid., p. 11.
37. Schellen, op. cit., p. 14.
38. Feversham Report, App. 1, paras 14–21.

39. David, G. and Lansac, J., 'The organisation of centers for the study and preservation of semen in France' in David and Price, pp. 15–26.
40. The Proceedings of the Symposium were published as David and Price.
41. Schoysman, R. and Schoysman-Deboeck, A.,'Present status of donor insemination in Belgium' in David and Price, pp. 27–30.
42. Campana et al., 'Present status of AID and sperm banks in Switzerland' in David and Price, pp. 35–9.
43. Lebech, P. E., 'Present status of AID and sperm banks in Denmark' in David and Price, pp. 41–4; for an earlier account see Feversham Report, App. 1, para. 43.
44. Traina, V., 'Artificial insemination and semen banks in Italy' in David and Price, pp. 51–8; for an earlier account see Feversham Report, App. 1, paras 30–5.
45. Marina, S. 'The first sperm bank in Spain: organisation and first year results' in David and Price, pp. 57–60; Portuando, J. A. and Echanojaurequi, A. D., 'Human semen bank at the Spanish Social Security Hospital' in David and Price, pp. 61–4.
46. Barkay, J. and Zuckerman H., 'AID and sperm bank development in Israel' in David and Price, pp. 45–50; for an earlier account see Feversham Report, App. 1, paras 26–9.
47. Rioux, J. E. and Ackman, C. D. F., 'Artificial insemination and sperm banks: the Canadian experience' in David and Price, pp. 31–4.
48. Caldwell, J. H., 'Babies by scientific selection', Scientific American (1934), 150, pp. 124–5.
49. Ploscowe, M., Sex and the Law (New York, Prentice-Hall, 1951), p. 113.
50. New York Post, 28 March 1955, pp. 4,18.
51. Lang, D., 'Artificial insemination: legitimate or illegitimate', McCall's Magazine (May 1955), p. 60.
52. Curie-Cohen et al., op. cit., p. 588.
53. 'Artificial Insemination of Married Women', 207 HL Deb., 5th ser., cols 926–1026; 26 February 1958, cols 934–5.
54. ibid., col. 957.
55. Feversham Report, para. 22.
56. e.g. Edwards, R. G., 'The current clinical and ethical situation of human conception in vitro' in Carter, C. O., ed., Developments in Human Reproduction and their Eugenic, Ethical Implications (London, Academic Press, 1983), pp. 53–116.
57. ibid., p. 95; BMA, 'Interim report on human in vitro fertilisation and embryo replacement and transfer', BMJ (1983), 226, pp. 1594–5; RCOG, 'Report of the RCOG Ethics Committee on in vitro fertilisation and embryo replacement or transfer', 1983.
58. Trounson, A. et al., 'Pregnancy established in an infertile patient after transfer of a donated embryo fertilised in vitro', BMJ (1983), 286, pp. 835–8.
59. 'Australia's wonder baby', The Times, 13 January 1984.
60. See Keane, N. and Breo, D., The Surrogate Mother. New York, Everest House, 1981. At least two American agencies now operate in the UK.

Chapter 4

1. IPPF, Handbook on Infertility, pp. 52–3; Stangel, op. cit., p. 157; Speichinger, J. P. and Maddox J. J., 'Homologous artificial insemination and oligospermia', Fert. & Ster. (1976), 27, pp. 135–8, at 135–6; Dixon, R. E. et al., 'Artificial insemination using homologous semen: a review of 158 cases', Fert. & Ster.

(1976), 27, pp. 647–54, at 647, Table 1; Guttmacher, A. F., 'Artificial insemination', *De Paul Law Rev.* (1969), 18, pp. 566–83, at 569; Foss, G. L. in RCOG (AI), pp. 44–5.

2. Dixon *et al.*, op. cit. (9.5% pregnancy rate.); Newton, J. R., RCOG (AI), p. 29 (results poor); Guttmacher A. F., 'The role of artificial insemination in the treatment of sterility', *Obs. & Gyn. Survey* (1960), 15, pp. 767–85 (success rate low).
3. IPPF, *Handbook*, pp. 52–3; Stangel, op. cit., p. 157; Speichinger and Maddox, op. cit., pp. 135–8; Dixon, R. E. and Buttram, V. C., 'Artificial insemination using donor semen: a review of 171 cases', *Fert. & Ster.* (1976), 27, pp. 130–4, at 130–1; Curie-Cohen, M. *et al.*, 'Current practice of artificial insemination by donor in the United States', *NEJM* (1979), 300, pp. 585–9, at 585–6; Behrman, S. J., 'Artificial insemination' in Behrman and Kistner, p. 783; Foss, G. L., 'Discussion opener' in RCOG (AI), pp. 44–5.
4. Sulewski, J. M. *et al.*, 'A longitudinal analysis of artificial insemination with donor semen', *Fert. & Ster.* (1978), 29, pp. 527–31.
5. ibid.
6. Behrman, S. J., 'Artificial insemination', *Fert. & Ster.* (1959), 10, pp. 248ff; Klugman, S. J., 'Therapeutic donor insemination', *Fert. & Ster.* (1954), 5, pp. 7ff; Portnoy, L., 'Artificial insemination (AID): experiences with its use in eighty barren marriages', *Fert. & Ster.* (1956), 7, pp. 327ff; Haman, J. O., 'Therapeutic donor insemination: a review of 440 cases', *Calif. Med.* (1959), 90, pp. 130ff; Steinberger, E. and Smith, K. D., 'Artificial insemination with fresh or frozen semen', *JAMA* (1973), 223, pp. 778ff; Hill, A. M., 'Experiences with artificial insemination' *Aust. & NZ J. Obs. & Gyn* (1970), 10, pp. 112ff; Slome, J., 'Artificial insemination by donor', *BMJ* (1973), 2, pp. 365–7.

Chapter 5

1. Clive, pp. 111–16; Bromley, p. 85; Clark, p. 60; also in Australia, see Finlay, H. A. and Bissett-Johnson, A., *Family Law in Australia* (Melbourne, Butterworths, 1972), p. 94; in South Africa, see Hahlo, H. R., *The South African Law of Husband and Wife* (Cape Town, Juta), p. 678.
2. Clive, p. 111; Bromley, p. 86.
3. Bromley, p. 87.
4. Clark, p. 685. In Australia wilful refusal is a ground of divorce, see Finlay and Bissett-Johnson, op. cit., pp. 307–8; and in South Africa it may amount to desertion, Hahlo, H. R., op. cit., p. 501.
5. Clive, p. 112.
6. *J. v. J.* 1978 SLT 128.
7. Clive, p. 111.
8. *D. v. A.* (1845), 1 Rob. Ecc. 279, at 298.
9. *Baxter v. Baxter* [1948] AC 274.
10. *Cowen v. Cowen* [1946], P 36 (Pilcher, J. held that penetration only was required, cf. du Parcq, L. J., at 40); see also *Grimes v. Grimes* [1948] P 323 (Finnemore, J. held that *coitus interruptus* is wilful refusal); cf. *White v. White* [1948] P 330, and *Cackett v. Cackett* [1950] P 253.
11. Bartholomew, G. P., 'Legal aspects of artificial insemination', *Mod. Law Rev.* (1958), 21, pp. 236–58, at 246.
12. *Corpus Iuris Secundum* (St Paul, Minn., West Publishing, 1974), 55, *sub nom.* 'Marriage', sec. 13, p. 826.
13. *T. v. M.* (1968) 100 NJ Super. 530; 242 A.2d. 670 (1968).
14. Clark, p. 113.
15. Uniform Marriage and Divorce Act s. 208(a)(2).

16. Hahlo, op. cit., p. 500.
17. Da Costa, op. cit., pp. 678ff.
18. Finlay and Bissett-Johnson, op. cit., pp. 94ff.
19. *Clarke v. Clarke* [1943] *2 All ER*, 540.
20. 1958 SC 105; 1958 SLT 12.
21. 1958 SC, at 113.
22. ibid.
23. Clive, pp. 53–7.
24. Bromley, p. 93 (approbation), now 'the petitioner's conduct' under the Matrimonial Causes Act 1973 s.13(1); Hahlo, op. cit., p. 491 (ratification); *Baxter v. Baxter*, op. cit. (acquiescence); *REL v. EL*, see n. 2 (estoppel).
25. *R.E.L. v. E.L.* [1949] P 211; *Slater v. Slater* [1953], P 235.
26. *The Church and the Law of Nullity of Marriage*. London, SPCK, 1955.
27. Cmnd. 9678.
28. Feversham Report.
29. *Family Law: nullity of marriage*, Working Paper no. 20. London, HMSO, 1968.
30. [1949] P 211.
31. [1953] P 235.
32. *The Times*, 12 May 1960.
33. *The Church and the Law of Nullity of Marriage*, op. cit.
34. Cmnd. 9678, para. 287.
35. Feversham Report, para. 108.
36. ibid., para. 156.
37. *Family Law: nullity of marriage*, op. cit., paras 37–42.
38. ibid., para. 42.
39. 1961 SC 347; also reported as *G. v. G.* 1961 SLT 324.
40. 1961 SC, at 349.
41. Hahlo, op. cit., p. 502.
42. Finlay and Bissett-Johnson, op. cit., p. 97.
43. Da Costa, op. cit., p. 680.
44. *Manbeck v. Manbeck*, 339 Pa Super 493; 489 A. 2d. 748 per Montemuro J.
45. 39 Misc. 2d 1083; 242 NYS 2d. 406 (1963).
46. Clive, p. 476.
47. Bromley, 5th edn, pp. 216–20.
48. Feversham Report, para. 73.
49. Divorce Reform Act 1969; now Matrimonial Causes Act 1973.
50. Divorce (Scotland) Act 1976.
51. Matrimonial Causes Act 1973 s.1 as amended by Matrimonial and Family Proceedings Act 1984; Divorce (Scotland) Act 1976 s.1.
52. Divorce (Scotland) Act 1976 s.1(3).
53. Matrimonial Causes Act 1973 s.2(5); Divorce (Scotland) Act 1976 s.2(2).
54. Matrimonial Causes Act 1973 s.1 as amended by Matrimonial and Family Proceedings Act 1984.
55. Divorce (Scotland) Act 1976 s.1(2)(b).
56. ibid., s.13(2).
57. Hahlo, op. cit., p. 373.
58. *Bell v. Bell* (1909) TS 500, at 508–9 per Innes, C. J.
59. Hahlo, op. cit., p. 373.
60. Finlay and Bissett-Johnson, op. cit., pp. 352ff.
61. Da Costa, op. cit., pp. 383ff.
62. see above.
63. Law Reform (Miscellaneous Provisions) Act 1949 s.4(1).
64. Krause, *Illegitimacy*, pp. 11–13.
65. Chapter 12.

Chapter 6

1. *Sapsford v. Sapsford* [1954] P 394, at 399.
2. Californian Civil Code s.93; other definitions can be found in New York Domestic Relations Law s.170; Georgia Code Ann. 30–102(6); Kansas Stat. Ann. 1970 Supp. 21–3507.
3. *Russell v. Russell* [1924] AC 687, at 721.
4. *Orford v. Orford* (1921) 59 DLR 251.
5. These cases are discussed later in the chapter.
6. Act 1563 c.10 'Anent Adulterie'.
7. Matt. 19:9; Cor. 7:13.
8. Lord Wheatley in *MacLennan v. MacLennan* 1958 SC 105, at 108.
9. *Hume's Lectures, I* (1766–1822) (Stair Society, vol. 5), 1939, 83.
10. Cretney, p. 107.
11. *First Report of the Commissioners into the Law of Divorce* (1853), C.1604.
12. ibid., para. 34.
13. Friedman, L. M., *A History of American Law* (New York, Simon & Schuster, 1973), pp. 179–84.
14. loc. cit.
15. loc. cit.
16. Rheinstein, M., *Marriage Stability, Divorce and the Law* (University of Chicago Press, 1972), ch. 4.
17. Slovenko, R., *Sexual Behaviour and the Law* (Illinois, Thomas, 1965), pp. 277ff.
18. 169 Wisc. 570 (1919).
19. Hill, G. B., ed., *Boswell's Life of Johnson* (Oxford, Clarendon Press, 1887), II, 55–6.
20. Russell, B., *Marriage and Morals* (London, Allen & Unwin, 1961), pp. 116–17.
21. Wangard, R. E., 'Artificial insemination and the law', *U. of Ill. Law Forum* (1968), pp. 203–31, at 217.
22. Westermarck, E., *The History of Human Marriage* (London, Macmillan, 1921), I, 299–36.
23. id., *The Origin and Development of the Moral Ideas* (London, Macmillan, 1906–8), II, 449–50.
24. Ellis, W. H., 'The socio-legal problems of artificial insemination', *Indiana Law Journal* (1953), 28, pp. 620–40, at 626.
25. Goode, W. J., *The Family* (New York, Prentice-Hall, 1963), ch. 1.
26. Harris, C. C., *The Family* (London, Allen & Unwin, 1969), pp. 53–4.
27. The Divorce Statistics produced by the Registrars General for Scotland, and England and Wales seem to suggest that there is a higher incidence of divorce among the childless. This has been challenged. See Chester, R., 'Is there a relationship between childlessness and marriage breakdown?', *J. BioSocial Science* (1971), 4, pp. 443–54.
28. Behrman, S. J., 'Artificial insemination' in Behrman and Kistner, pp. 779–89, at 781.
29. Muller, H. J., 'Genetic progress by voluntarily conducted germinal choice' in Wolstenholme, G., ed., *Man and his Future*. Ciba Foundation Symposium. London, Churchill, 1963.
30. *Los Angeles Times*, 29 February 1980.
31. *New York Times*, 11 December 1985.
32. *Sunday Times*, 21 August 1983.
33. (1921) 58 DLR 251.
34. *Hoch v. Hoch* (1945), Unreported 1945 no. 44-C-9307, Cir. Ct., Cook Co., Ill.
35. *Doornbos v. Doornbos* (1954), Unreported no. 54-S-14981 Sup. Ct. Cook Co., Ill. Appeal 12 Ill. App 2d 473; 139 N.E. 2d 844 (1956).

36. *People v. Sorensen*, 437 P. 2d. 495; 66 Cal. Rep. 285; 68 Cal. Rep. 7 (1968).
37. *MacLennan v. MacLennan* 1958 SC 105; 1958 SLT 12.
38. Dickens, B., *Medico-Legal Aspects of Family Law* (Toronto, Butterworths, 1979), p. 7.
39. Chandler, H. S., 'A legislative approach to artificial insemination', *Cornell LR* (1968), 53, pp. 497–513, at 502; Sergeant, D. A., 'Legal status of artificial insemination: a need for policy formulation', *Drake LR* (1970), 19, pp. 409–40, at 420–1.
40. Jacobs, R. S. and Luedtke, J. P., 'Social and legal aspects of human artificial insemination', *Wisconsin LR* (1965), 40, pp. 859–84, at 833–4; Sherman, J. S., 'People v. Sorensen: artificial insemination gives birth to legal problems in California', *Calif. Western LR* (1968), 4, pp. 177–98, at 198.

Chapter 7

1. 190 Misc. 786; 78 NYS 2d, 390 (1948).
2. No. 54, s.14891 Super ct. Cook Co.: On Appeal 12 Ill 2d, 473; 139 NE 2d 1844 (1956).
3. 15 Misc. 2d. 260 (1958).
4. 39 Misc. 2d. 1083; 242 NYS 2d. 406 (1963).
5. 41 Misc. 2d. 886; 246 NYS 2d. 835 (1964).
6. 68 C. 2d. 280 (1968).
7. s.7 as amended by Family Law (Scotland) Act 1985 Sch. 1.
8. ss 41; 52.
9. ss 1, 88.
10. s.1.
11. Geo. Stat. 74–101: la (Supp. 1970).
12. s. 1. The Act applies to deaths after 31 March 1976.
13. Family Law Reform Act 1969 s.15(1); Law Reform (Miscellaneous Provisions) (Scotland) Act 1968 s.5.

Chapter 8

1. Adoption Act 1976 (England & Wales); Adoption (Scotland) Act 1978.
2. Graveson, R. H., *Status in the Common Law* (London, Athlone Press, 1953), p. 2.
3. 'Marriage, as understood in Christendom, may for this purpose be defined as the voluntary union for life of one man and one woman to the exclusion of all others', *Hyde v. Hyde* (1866) LR 1 P & D 130, at 133; Friedmann, W., *Law in a Changing Society*, 2nd edn (Harmondsworth, Penguin, 1972), p. 281.
4. (UK) Stair, *The Institutions of the Law of Scotland*, 5th edn, ed. More, J. S. (Edinburgh, Bell & Bradfute, 1832), III, 3, p. 42; Blackstone, W., *Commentaries on the Laws of England*, ed. Kerr, R. M. (London, Murray, 1862), I, 460; (USA) Krause, *Family Law*, p. 14.
5. *S. v. S.; W. v. Official Solicitor* [1972] AC 24, at 45.
6. In some jurisdictions children of void and voidable marriages may be legitimate (US, UK, France, West Germany, The Netherlands, Switzerland) and polygamous marriages may be recognized (US, UK, Australia). In the US case of *Levy v. Louisiana* 391 US 68 (1968) the Supreme Court declared invalid a 'wrongful death' statute which purported to bar recovery by a mother for the death of her unacknowledged illegitimate child.
7. UK (England & Wales), Cretney, pp. 577–80; (Scotland) Clive, p. 182; USA,

Krause, *Family Law*, pp. 799–836; also Canada, Divorce Act s.2.10; France, Civil Code Art. 312; West Germany, Civil Code Art. 1593; The Netherlands, Civil Code Art. 205.

8. UK (Scotland), Stair, III, 3, 42; (England) Blackstone, p. 460; USA, Krause, *Illegitimacy*, pp. 15–17.

9. Smith, George P. II, 'Through a test tube darkly: artificial insemination and the law', *Michigan* (1968–9), 67, pp. 127–50; Walker, D. M., *Principles of Scottish Private Law*, 3rd edn (Oxford University Press, 1983), p. 293.

10. Smith, op. cit., p. 134.

11. e.g. The Netherlands, Civil Code Art. 201:1; Switzerland, Civil Code Art. 256(3).

12. *People ex rel Abajian v. Dennett*, 184 NYS 2d. 178 at 183; 15 Misc. 2d. 260 at 264 (1958). A similar decision was reached in the unreported case of *Ohlsen v. Ohlsen* (1954), Sup. Ct., Cook Co., Ill.

13. Chappel, A., 'Artificial insemination', *J. American Medical Women's Assoc.* (1959), 14, pp. 901–4; Foss, G. L. in RCOG (AI), p. 45; Guttmacher, A. F., 'The role of artificial insemination in the treatment of sterility', *Obs. & Gyn. Survey* (1960), 15, pp. 767–85, at 777.

14. This practice is probably less common today. See Curie-Cohen, M. *et al.*, 'Current practice of artificial insemination by donor in the United States', *NEJM* (1979), 300, pp. 585–90, at 587; Newton, J. in RCOG (AI), p. 55.

15. Newton, J. R., 'Current status of AI in clinical practice' in RCOG (AI), pp. 25–39, at 37; Behrman, S. J., 'Artificial insemination' in Behrman and Kistner, pp. 779–89, at 785.

16. Jacob, J., ed., *Speller's Law Relating to Hospitals*, 6th edn (London, H. K. Lewis, 1978), ch. 20.

17. 190 Misc. 786; 78 NYS 2d 390 (Sup. Ct. 1948).

18. 190 Misc., at 787–8; 78 NYS, 2d, at 391–2.

19. No. 54–5 – 12981 (Super. Ct. Cook Co. 1954) (unreported); Appeal 12, Ill. App. 2d 473; 139 Ne 2d 844 (1956).

20. The opinion of the trial judge is quoted in Levisohn, A. A., 'Dilemma in parenthood', *J. For. Med.* (1957), 4, pp. 147–72, at 162.

21. 39 Misc. 2d 1083; 242 NYS, 2d. 406 (1963).

22. 39 Misc. 2d, at 1085; 242 NYS, 2d, at 408.

23. *In re Adoption of Anonymous*, 74 Misc. 2d. 99; 345 NYS, 2d, 430 (1973).

24. New York Domestic Relations Law 1969 s.24.

25. 74 Misc. 2d, at 104–5; 345 NYS, 2d, at 435–6.

26. 66 Cal. Rep. 7; 437 p.2d 495; 68 Cal. Rep. 685 (1968).

27. *Roberts v. Roberts* (1971) VR 160.

28. *V. v. R.* (1979) (3) SA 1006.

29. Matrimonial Causes Act 1973 s.52(1); Matrimonial Proceedings (Children) Act 1958 s.7 (Scotland), as amended by Family Law (Scotland) Act 1985 s.1.

30. Matrimonial Causes Act 1973 s.27(1); Domestic Proceedings and Magistrates' Courts Act 1978 s.2(1).

31. Inheritance (Provision for Family and Dependants) Act 1975 s.1(1).

32. Weinstock, N., 'Artificial insemination – the problem and the solution', *Family Law Quarterly* (1971), 5, pp. 369–402, at 391–7; Wangard, R. E., 'Artificial insemination and the law', *University of Illinois Law Forum* (1968), pp. 203–31, at 229–31; Chandler, H. S., 'Legislative approach to artificial insemination', *Cornell L.R.* (1968), 53, pp. 487–513, at 512–13; Sergeant, D. A., 'Legal status of artificial insemination: a need for policy formulation', *Drake L.R.* (1970), 9, pp. 409–440, at 438–440; Sherman, J. S., 'People v. Sorensen: artificial insemination gives birth to real problems in California', *California Western LR* (1986), 4, pp. 177–98, at 195–8; Wadlington, W., 'Arti-

ficial insemination: the dangers of a poorly kept secret', *North Western University LR* (1970), 64, pp. 777–807, at 803–7; Klayman, E. T., 'Therapeutic impregnation: prognosis of a lawyer – diagnosis of a legislature', *University of Cincinnati LR* (1970), 39, pp. 291–330, at 325–30; Thompson, C. M., 'The legal consequences of artificial insemination in South Dakota', *South Dakota* (1968), 13, pp. 171–81, at 179–81. Rice, C. E., 'AID: an heir of controversy', *Notre Dame Lawyer* (1959), 34, pp. 510–29; Dienes, C. T., 'Artificial donor insemination: perspectives on legal and social change', *Iowa LR* (1968), 54, pp. 253–317, at 315–17; Ellis, W. H., 'The socio-legal problems of artificial insemination', *Indiana Law Journal* (1953), 28, pp. 620–40, at 634–40.

Bills were introduced in several states in the United States making express provision whereby the AID child would have been regarded as legitimate: Indiana House Bill 350 (1949); New York Senate Bill 745 (1948); New York Senate Bill 772 (1949); New York Senate Bill 579 (1950); New York Senate Bill 493 (1951); Virginia Senate Bill 199 (1948); Wisconsin Assembly Bill 407 (1949). Three Bills were introduced in Minnesota: House Bills 1090, 1091 and 1092 (all of 1949). The first of these prohibited all artificial insemination, the second prohibited only AID, but the third permitted both AIH and AID under certain conditions. In 1955 a Bill was introduced into the Ohio Legislature (Ohio Senate Bill 93) which would have made the practice of AID a crime by the doctor and the woman, and any child born as the result would have been illegitimate. All these Bills were unsuccessful. More recently proposals have been made in Alberta (Alberta Institute of Law Research *Status of Children*, Report no. 20, 1976); 9th Report of the Royal Commission on Family and Children's Law, British Columbia. Bills have been introduced in the UK and France and a draft Recommendation has come from the Council of Europe.

Senator Charles A. Root who introduced the three Bills in Minnesota recorded some of the reaction in a letter to the author of an article on artificial insemination: 'Extensive hearings were had on all three Bills. Lobbying against the Bills was terrific. Most of the lobbyists made no distinction between the provisions of the three bills. Certain religious groups became quite fanatical on the subject. The personal abuse that I and members of my family took was unbelievable. Vicious, anonymous calls were received by the hundreds. No member of my family was spared. For a considerable period it was impossible for my children to run errands to the various centres or otherwise venture on the streets. In all the twelve years that I have served on the Legislature, I have never seen anything that would compare with the hearings in connection with these bills. My correspondence was so heavy that I had to hire one girl who did nothing else except answer my correspondence with respect to these bills.' See Shell, Thurston A., 'Artificial insemination – legal and related problems', *U. Fla. L.R.* (1955), 8, p. 315.

33. Social Trends (1986), Table 2.26.
34. Population Trends 14 (1978) (HMSO), p. 15; see also Population Trends 30 (1982), pp. 9–14.
35. Rheinstein, M., *Marriage, Stability, Divorce and the Law*. University of Chicago Press, 1972.
36. Social Trends (1986), Table 1.11.
37. Apart from the USA and the UK (see n. 4 above) the following countries have provisions dealing with the children of void and voidable marriages, and in certain circumstances these children are declared legitimate: France, West Germany, The Netherlands, Switzerland, Spain, USSR, Poland, Sweden, Yugoslavia, Czechoslovakia, Australia, India.

38. Gloag, W. M. and Henderson, R. C., *Introduction to the Law of Scotland*, 8th edn (Edinburgh, W. Green, 1980), pp. 748–9, Legitimacy Act 1976 s.1(1).
39. Law Reform (Miscellaneous Provisions) Act 1949 s.4(1).
40. Krause, *Illegitimacy*, pp. 11–14.
41. Feversham Report, Memo of Dissent, para. 14.
42. AID Children (Legal Status) Bill 1977. The Bill failed to secure a second reading because of pressure of parliamentary time.
43. Feversham Report, para. 170.
44. Adoption (Scotland) Act 1978 s.45(5); Adoption Act 1976 s.5D (E. & W.).
45. Snowden and Mitchell, pp. 82ff.
46. Dunstan, G. R., 'Ethical issues relating to AID' in RCOG (AI), pp. 185–7.
47. Lord Kilbrandon in Ciba, p. 93.
48. Cusine, D. J., 'Status of the AID child', *SLT* (News) (1977), pp. 161–2, at 162.
49. It was suggested by the Royal Commission on Marriage and Divorce 1956, Cmnd 9678, para. 393, for the purposes of 'matrimonial disputes' and was implemented in the Matrimonial Proceedings (Children) Act 1958 s.7. It is also recognized for the purposes of social security (see Child Benefit Act 1975 s.2) and for income tax (Income and Corporation Taxes Act 1970 s. 10).
50. Matrimonial Causes Act 1973 s.52(1); Matrimonial Proceedings (Children) Act 1958 s.7.
51. Inheritance (Provision for Family and Dependants) Act 1975 s.1.
52. USA: Krause, *Illegitimacy*, pp. 13–14, 19–21; France: Civil Code, arts. 335–9; West Germany: Civil Code, art. 1600: *The Netherlands*: Civil Code, arts. 221–4.
53. Wangard, R. E., 'Artificial insemination and the law', *University of Illinois Law Forum* (1968), pp. 203–31, esp. at 228; Chandler, Hardy S., 'Legislative approach to artificial insemination', *Cornell L.R.* (1968), 53, pp. 497–513, esp. at 498; Sherman, J. S., 'People v. Sorensen: artificial insemination gives birth to legal problems in California', *California Western LR* (1968), 4, pp. 177–98, esp. at 194.
54. Georgia Code Ann. 74–101.1.
55. Oklahoma Statutes Ann. Title 10 551–53 (1967) (Supp 1968).
56. Alaska Stat. s.20.20.010 (1975).
    California Civil Code s.7005 (West. Supp. 1982).
    Colorado Rev. Stat. s.19–6406 (1978).
    Connecticut Gen. Stat. s.45–69 f-n (1981).
    Florida Stat. S742.11 (West Supp. 1982).
    Georgia Code, Ann. S 19–7–21 (1982).
    Idaho Code S 39–5401–5407 (Supp 1982).
    Kansas Stat. Ann. s.23–129 (1981).
    Louisiana Civil Code Ann Art 118 (West Supp 1982).
    Maryland Est. and Trust Code Ann s.1–206 (1974).
    Massachussets Gen. Laws ch. 46 s.4b (West Supp 82–3).
    Michigan Comp. Law s.700–1111(2) (1979).
    Minnesota Stat. s.257.56 (1980).
    Montana Code, Ann. s.40–6–106 (1981).
    Nevada Rev. Stat. s.126.061 (1983).
    New York Domestic Relation Law s.73 (McKinney, 1977).
    North Carolina Gen. Stat. s.49A–1 (1976).
    Oklahoma Stat. tit. 10 s.552 (1981).
    Oregon Rev. Stat. 109.243 (1981).
    Tennesse Code, Ann. S.53–446 (Supp. 1982).
    Texas Code, Ann. 12–03.
    Virginia Code S.64.1–7.1 (1980).

Washington Rev. Code s.26,26.050 (1981).
Wisconsin Stat. s.891.40 (1979–80).
Wyoming Stat. Ann. s.14–2.103 (1978).
57. The Uniform Parentage Act was promulgated in 1973 by the National Council of Commissioners on Uniform State Laws and approved by the House of Delegates of the American Bar Association in 1974.
58. Kansas Stat. Ann.23–128–130 (Supp. 1973).
59. Oregon Laws 1977, ch. 686 s.3(1).
60. Weinstock, N., 'Artificial insemination: the problem and the solution', *Family Law Quarterly* (1971), 5, pp. 369–402, at 395.
61. Law Commission, *Family Law: illegitimacy* (London, HMSO, 1982), paras 12.16–17.
62. Portuguese Civil Code, art.1799; Swiss Civil Code, art. 256(3); Dutch Civil Code, art. 201.1.
63. SFS 1984; 12140, which came into force 18 March 1985.
64. The Draft Recommendation was amended by the European Committee on Legal Co-operation at its 30th Meeting (27 November–1 December 1978) and by the European Public Health Committee at its 6th Meeting (13–16 November 1979). A final draft dealing with Artificial Procreation was approved in April 1987 for submission to the Council of Ministers in December 1987.

Chapter 9

1. In Israel in 1979 the Director General of the Ministry of Health issued 'Rules Concerning the Administration of Sperm Banks and Directives for the Performance of Artificial Insemination'. Rule 26 provides: 'The identity of the donor, on the one hand, and that of the husband and wife on the other hand, may be revealed to no one, including either party.' Guidelines issued in 1981 by the Senate of the Swiss Academy of Medical Sciences has a similar provision (Guideline 5). In neither case is a penalty for disclosure specified.
2. Veatch, R. M., *Case Studies in Medical Ethics* (Cambridge, Mass., Harvard University Press, 1977), pp. 116–18.
3. s. 21: 07 (1959).
4. Slovenia: Law of 21 April 1977 s.36; Croatia: Law of 21 April 1978, art. 32.
5. Examples are Colorada: Rev. Stat. Ann. 19–6–106 (1978); Connecticut: Gen. Stat. Ann. 45–69f (1980); Kansas: Stat. Ann. s.23–128 (1971); Oklahoma; Rev. Stat. Ann: tit. 10, 553 (1971).
6. Medical Act 1983 s.36 (UK).
7. ibid.
8. See 'General Medical Council: Disciplinary Committee', *BMJ* Supp. (1971), pp. 79–80.
9. Holder, A. R., *Medical Malpractice Law*, 2nd edn (New York, Wiley, 1978), pp. 273–4.
10. Mich. Stat. Ann. s.14–533.
11. French Penal Code, art. 378; Dutch Civil Code, art. 272(1); Italian Penal Code, art. 622.
12. New Zealand, Victoria, Tasmania, Newfoundland, Great Britain, USA Model Code and Proposed Federal Rules.
13. e.g. The National Health Service (Venereal Disease) Regs. 1974 SI. 1974/29 Reg. 2.
14. Holder, op. cit., pp. 1–7.
15. ibid., p. 273.

16. ibid., pp. 398–408.
17. *Pfizer Corporation v. Ministry of Health* [1965] AC 512.
18. *The Times*, 28 March 1896.
19. *Att. Gen. v. Mulholland and Foster* [1963] 2 QB. 477.
20. [1967] 2 All ER 415.
21. *AB v. CD* (1851) 14 D. 177.
22. *AB v. CD* (1904) 7 F. 72.
23. Working Paper no. 58, 'Confidential information' (1974); Memorandum no. 40, 'Confidential information' (1977).
24. Holder, op. cit., pp. 273–7; Fiscina, S., 'Information about patients: how confidential?' *Legal Medicine* (1980), pp. 247–60.
25. Fiscina, S., op. cit., pp. 247–8.
26. ibid., p. 248.
27. e.g. *Vigil v. Rice*, 397 P. 2d 719 (1964).
28. See below.
29. See below.
30. Rubin, B., 'Psychological aspects of human artificial insemination', *Arch. Gen. Psychiat.* (1965), 13, pp. 121–31, at 129.
31. Goldstein, J., Freud, A. and Solnit, A., *Beyond the Best Interests of the Child* (New York, Free Press, 1973), pp. 16–17.
32. Stat. Ann. s.23–129 (Supp. 1971).
33. Raynor, L., *The Adopted Child Comes of Age* (London, Allen & Unwin, 1980), pp. 127, 132, 146, 148.
34. Triselotis, J., 'Identity and adoption', *Child Adoption* (1974), 78, pp. 27–34; Raynor, op. cit., pp. 90–4.
35. Sants, H. J., 'Genealogical bewilderment in children with substitute parents', *Brit. J. Med. Psych.* (1964), 37, pp. 133–41; Triselotis, J., *In Search of Origins: the experience of adopted people*. London, Routledge, 1973.
36. Adoption (Scotland) Act 1978 s.45(5); Adoption Act 1976 s.51(2).
37. Adoption (Scotland) Act 1978 s.45(1); Adoption Act 1976 s.51.
38. Klibanoff, E. B., 'Genealogical information in adoption', *Family Law Quarterly* (1977), 11, pp. 185–98, at 187; note 'The adoptee's right to know its natural heritage', *New York Law Forum* (1973), 19, pp. 137–56.
39. 'Sealed adoption records vs. the adoptee's right to know the identity of his birth parents', *Children's Rights Report* (1979), III, no. 5 (February), p. 2.
40. e.g. Kansas: Stat. Ann. s.65–2423 (1972) and Supp. 1979.
41. Virginia Code s.63–1–236 (1973).
42. *Children's Rights Report*, op. cit., p. 6.
43. e.g. New York Domestic Relations Law s.114.
44. *In re Ann Carol S, NYLJ*, 31 (1974).
45. *Lovallo v. NJ State Register*, 148 NJ Super 302 (1977).
46. *McGowan v. Maryland*, 366 US 420 (1961).
47. *Reed v. Reed*, 404 US 71 (1971).
48. *Frontiero v. Richardson* 411 US 677 at 686 (1973).
49. *Weber v. Aetna Casualty and Surety Co.*, 406 US 164 (1972); but see *Jimenez v. Weinberger* 417 US 628 (1974).
50. Ploscowe, M., 'The place of law in medico-moral problems: a legal view', *NYULR* (1956), 31, pp. 1238–45, at 1243.
51. Kelly, H. A., 'Kinship, incest and the dictates of law', *Am. J. Juris* (1969), 14, pp. 69–78, at 78.
52. Feversham Report, para. 39.
53. Moser, W., 'Population genetics and AID', and Jacquard, A. and Schoevaeri, D., 'Artificial insemination and consanguinity' in David and Price, pp. 379–83; 385–7.

54. Feversham Report, para. 39.
55. ibid., para. 216.
56. This point was made by Curie-Cohen *et al.* in their survey, 'Current practice of artificial insemination by donor in the United States', *NEJM* (1979), 300, pp. 585–90.
57. Snowden and Mitchell; Snowden, Mitchell and Snowden.
58. SFS 1984: 1140, which came into force 18 March 1985.
59. *Children Conceived by Artificial Insemination* (SOU, 1983: 42).

Chapter 10

1. Feversham Report, para. 33.
2. Guttmacher, A. F., 'The role of artificial insemination in the treatment of human sterility', *Bull. NY Academy of Science* (1943), 119, pp. 573–91, at 588.
3. Joyce, D., 'Recruitment, selection and matching of donors' in RCOG (AI), pp. 60–8, at 60; Saunders, D. M., 'The assessment of the infertile couple for AID', in Wood, p. 49.
4. Joyce, op. cit., p. 60; Goldstein, D. P., 'Artificial insemination by donor: status and problems' in Milunsky, A. and Annas, G. J., eds, *Genetics and the Law*. New York, Plenum Press, 1976.
5. Guttmacher, A. F., 'Artificial insemination', *De Paul Law Rev.* (1969), 18, pp. 566–83, at 571.
6. Joyce, op. cit., p. 61.
7. Rioux, J. E. and Ackman, C. D. F., 'Artificial insemination and sperm banks: the Canadian experience' in David and Price, pp. 31–4.
8. Marina, S., 'The first sperm bank in Spain: organisation and first year results' in David and Price, pp. 57–60.
9. Curie-Cohen, M. *et al.*, 'Current practice of artificial insemination by donor in the United States', *NEJM* (1979), 300, pp. 585–90.
10. Weisman, A. I., 'Selection of donors for use in artificial insemination', *West. J. Surg.* (1942), 50, pp. 142–4.
11. Johnston, I., 'The donor' in Wood, p. 13.
12. David, G. and Lansac, J., 'The organisation of the centers for the study and preservation of semen in France' in David and Price, pp. 15–26, at 20.
13. *Handbook on Infertility* (London, IPPF, 1979), p. 50.
14. Schoysman, R., 'Problems of selecting donors for AI', *J. Med. Eth.* (1975), 1, pp. 34–5.
15. Marina, S., op. cit., p. 57.
16. 'Rules concerning the Administration of Sperm Banks and Directives for the Performance of Artificial Insemination' (1979), ch. 3, Rule 27(iv).
17. Dawkins, R., *The Selfish Gene* (Oxford University Press, 1976), p. 151.
18. Feversham Report, para. 34.
19. David, G. and Lansac, J., op. cit., p. 20.
20. The Draft Recommendation was approved by the Committee on Legal Co-operation at its 30th Meeting (27 November–1 December 1978) and by the Public Health Committee at its 6th Meeting (13–16 November 1979). A final draft dealing with artificial procreation will be submitted to the Council of Ministers in October 1987.
21. BMA Panel, para. 27.
22. Feversham Report, App. 1, para. 45; Curie-Cohen *et al.*, op. cit., p. 587.
23. Johnston, I., op. cit., p. 13 (Australia); Rioux, J. E. and Ackman, C. D. F., op. cit., p. 32 (Canada). The Law Reform Commission in Ontario

recommends that donors should be paid only reasonable expenses (Recommendation 15,1).

24. Marina, S., op. cit., p. 58 (Spain); Lebech, P. E. and Detlefsen, G., 'Artificial insemination with frozen spermatozoa: results from 1967 to 1978' in David and Price, pp. 249–57, at 250 (Denmark).
25. Annas, G. J., 'Artificial insemination: beyond the best interests of the donor', *Hastings Center Report* (1979), 9, no. 4, pp. 14–15, 43, at 14.
26. Titmus, R., *The Gift Relationship*. New York, Pantheon, 1971.
27. Annas, op. cit., p. 14.
28. *Carter v. Inter Faith Hospital of Queens*, 60 Misc 2d. 733 (1969).
29. *Perlmutter v. Beth David Hospital*, 308 NY 100; 123 NE 2d. 792 (1954).
30. Walker, D. M., *Principles of Scottish Private Law*, 3rd edn (Oxford University Press, 1983), pp. 125–6; Hahlo, H. R. and Kahn, E., *The Union of South Africa: the development of its laws and constitution* (London, Stevens, 1965), pp. 487–90.
31. Treitel, G. H., *The Law of Contract*, 6th edn. (London, Stevens, 1979), ch. 15 (England).
32. Joyce, op. cit., p. 63; Johnston, op. cit., p. 15; Dixon, R. E. and Buttram, V. C., 'Artificial insemination using donor semen: a review of 171 cases' *Fert. & Ster.* (1976), 27, pp. 130–4, at 131; Curie-Cohen *et al.*, op. cit., p. 586; Behrman, S. J., 'Artificial insemination' in Behrman and Kistner, pp. 779–89, at 785.
33. For such a list see Snowden and Mitchell, p. 64.
34. *The Times*, 20 November 1984.
35. ibid., 14 September 1985.
36. RCOG (AI), p. 65.
37. ibid., p. 61.
38. ibid., p. 64; Johnston, op. cit., p. 14.
39. Johnston, ibid.
40. Curie-Cohen, op. cit., p. 585.
41. David, and Lansac, J., op. cit., p. 20.
42. Joyce, op. cit., pp. 64–5.
43. Fiumara, N. J., 'Transmission of gonorrhea by artificial insemination', *Brit. J. Venereal Diseases* (1972), 48, pp. 308–9.
44. Sherman, J. K. and Rosenfeld, J., 'Importance of frozen-stored human semen in the spread of gonorrhea', *Fert. & Ster.* (1975), 26, pp. 1043–7; Smith, R. S. and Tagatz, G. E., 'Acute gonorrhea after artificial insemination', *Fert. & Ster.* (1976), 27, pp. 1338–9.
45. Johnston, op. cit., p. 15.
46. David and Lansac, op. cit., p. 20.
47. Campana, A. *et al.*, 'Present status of AID and sperm banks in Switzerland' in David and Price, pp. 35–9, at 35; Marina, S., op. cit., p. 58.
48. A very readable account of this complex topic is in Jones, A. and Bodmer, W. F., *Our Future Inheritance: choice or chance?* (Oxford University Press, 1974), pp. 45–82.
49. Curie-Cohen *et al.*, op. cit., p. 588.
50. Edwards, J. H., 'Discussion Opener on Mr Joyce's paper' in RCOG (AI), p. 72 (against karyotyping); Johnston, op. cit., p. 15 (against karyotyping). The following use karyotyping: Rioux, J. E. and Ackman, C. D. F., op. cit., p. 32; Campana, A. *et al.*, op. cit., p. 36; Portuando, J. A. and Echanojaurequi, A. D., 'Human semen bank at the Spanish Social Security Hospital' in David and Price, pp. 61–4, at 62; David, G. *et al.*, 'Results of AID for a first and succeeding pregnancies' in ibid., pp. 211–21, at 212.
51. Sherman, J. K., 'Synopsis of the use of human frozen semen since 1964: state of the art of human semen banking', *Fert. & Ster.* (1973), 24, pp. 397–412.

52. Oregon Rev. Stat. s.677.360 (1977) s.5.
53. Law, 21 April 1977, Part IV s.34.
54. Law, 21 April 1978, Part IV art. 33.
55. New York City Health Code 1959, Artificial Human Insemination, 21.05.
56. Rules, op. cit., ch. 3, Rule 27.
57. 'Schweizerische Aerztezeitung', *Bulletin des Medecins Suisses* (1982), 62, no. 11, p. 623.
58. Foss, G. L., 'Discussion opener' in RCOG (AI), p. 44.
59. Joyce, op. cit., p. 68; Johnston, op. cit., p. 18.
60. Edwards, J. H., 'Discussion opener', op. cit., p. 70.
61. *Pfizer Corporation v. Ministry of Health* (1965) AC 512.
62. Walker, D. M., *The Law of Delict in Scotland*, 2nd edn. (Edinburgh, Green, 1982), pp. 173–207; Clerk, J. F. and Lindsell, W. H., *The Law of Torts*, 15th edn. (London, Sweet & Maxwell, 1974), para. 10.01ff; Prosser, W. L., *Handbook of the Law of Torts*, 6th edn. (St Paul, Minn., West Pub., 1971), ch. 2.
63. Descriptions collected by Greer, L. J. in *Hall v. Brooklands Auto-Racing Club* [1933] 1 KB, 205, at 224.
64. *Bolam v. Friern Hospital Management Committee* [1957] 2 All E.R. 118, per McNair, J., at 127; *Whitehouse v. Jordan* [1981] 1 All E.R. 267.
65. Prosser, op. cit., p. 162.
66. Walker, op. cit., pp. 169–73; Clerk and Lindsell, op. cit., ch. 1; Prosser, op. cit., p. 143.
67. Curie-Cohen *et al.*, op. cit., p. 588.
68. *Hunter v. Hanley* 1955 SC 200, per Lord President Clyde, at 204–5.
69. 63 Mich. App. 79; 234 N.W. 2d 411 (1975).
70. Walker, op. cit., pp. 207–31; Clerk and Lindsell, op. cit., para. 1.111–1.115; Prosser, op. cit., p. 143–5; Hart, H. L. A. and Honoré, A. M., *Causation in the Law* (Oxford, Clarendon Press, 1959), *passim*.
71. s. 1.
72. *Report on Injuries to Unborn Children*. Cmnd 5709 (1974).
73. *Liability for Ante-Natal Injury*. Cmnd 5371 (1973).
74. *Royal Commission on Civil Liability and Compensation for Personal Injuries*. Cmnd 7054–1 (HMSO, 1974), chs 9–11, 17.
75. New Zealand Compensation Act 1974, discussed in *Royal Commission on Civil Liability etc.*, op. cit., paras 219–29.

Chapter 11

1. Eliason, R., 'Assessment of male fertility' in RCOG (AI), pp. 142–50; Mattei, A. *et al.*, 'The male factor in AID requests', in David and Price, pp. 313–24.
2. Behrman, S. J. and Kistner, R. W., 'A rational approach to the evaluation of infertility' in Behrman and Kistner, pp. 1–14, esp. p. 6 (10m/ml); Saunders, D. M., 'The assessment of the infertile couple for AID' in Wood, pp. 38–49 (most clinics accept 18m/ml); Guttmacher, A. F., 'The role of artificial insemination in the treatment of human sterility', *Bull. NY Academy of Science* (1943), 119, pp. 573–91 (30m/ml).
3. *Skinner v. Oklahoma* 316 US 535 (1942) gives limited protection against state action which attempts to interfere with a person's capacity to procreate.
4. art. 12.
5. *Skinner v. Oklahoma*, op. cit., considered the constitutionality of a statute which made provision for the sterilization of certain types of criminals.
6. *Eisenstadt v. Baird* 405 US 438 (1972); *Carey v. Population Services International*

431 US 678 (1977). The US Supreme Court held that statutes which restricted the distribution of contraceptives were unconstitutional.

7. Clerk, J. F. and Lindsell, W. F., *The Law of Torts*, 15th edn (London, Sweet & Maxwell, 1982), 10.48–10.51; Walker, D. M., *The Law of Delict in Scotland*, 2nd edn. Edinburgh, W. Green, 1981; Prosser, W. L., *Handbook of the Law of Torts*, 6th edn (St Paul, Minn., West Pub., 1976), p. 63.

8. e.g. *Ravenis v. Detroit General Hospital* 63 Mich. App. 79; 234 NW. 2d. 411 (1975).

9. e.g. *Dumer v. St Michael's Hospital* 69 Wisc. 2d. 233; 233 NW. 2d 372, (1975) Sup. Ct. Wisconsin; *Chatterton v. Gerson and anr* [1981], 1 All ER 257.

10. Jones, A. and Bodmer, W. F., *Our Future Inheritance: choice or chance?* (Oxford University Press, 1974), p. 52.

11. *Dumer v. St Michael's Hospital*, op. cit.

12. *McKay v. Essex Health Authority* [1982] 2 All ER 771.

13. Saunders, op. cit.

14. Professor A. I. Klopper, University of Aberdeen. Personal communication.

15. Behrman, S. J., 'Artificial insemination' in Behrman and Kistner, pp. 779–89, at 785; Dixon, R. E. and Buttram, V. C., 'Artificial insemination using donor semen: a review of 171 cases', *Fert. & Ster.* (1976), 27, pp. 130–4, at 133; Rioux, J. E. and Ackman, C. D. F., 'Artificial insemination and sperm banks in Canada' in David and Price, pp. 31–4; Bremond, A. *et al.*, 'Evaluation of female fertility before AID' in David and Price, pp. 325–31; Kerr, M. and Templeton, A., 'Selection and counselling of recipients' in RCOG (AI), pp. 80–5, at 81.

16. Saunders, op. cit., pp. 48–9.

17. *Whitehouse v. Jordon* [1981] 1 All ER 267 (HL).

18. Chamberlain, G. and Brown, J. C., 'Complication of laparoscopy' in *Gynaecological Laparoscopy*. Report of the Working Party of the Confidential Inquiry into Gynaecological Laparoscopy (RCOG, 1978), pp. 105–39.

19. Jacob, J. ed., *Speller's Law Relating to Hospitals and Kindred Institutions*, 6th edn (London, H. K. Lewis, 1978), ch. 13; Holder, A. R., *Medical Malpractice Law*, 2nd edn (New York, Wiley, 1978), *passim*.

20. Jacob, loc. cit.; Mason, J. K. and McCall-Smith, A. A., *Law and Medical Ethics* (London, Butterworths, 1983), ch. 9.

21. Jacob, op. cit., pp. 192–202; *Gillick v. West Norfolk and Wisbech Area Health Authority* [1985] 3 All ER 402 (HL) (England & Wales); Holder, op. cit., ch. 1.

22. Jacob, op. cit., pp. 204–6; Mental Health Act 1983 ss. 56–64; Mental Health (Scotland) Act 1984 s.96; Holder, op. cit., p. 247.

23. Jacob, op. cit., pp. 204–6; Holder, op. cit., pp. 243–4.

24. *Bravery v. Bravery* [1954] 1 WLR 1169, at 1180.

25. Jacob, op. cit., pp. 203–4.

26. One obstetrician has said that it is justifiable to provide AID for a married woman without the husband's consent where the husband is sterile but might be hurt if he was told of his condition. Loveset, J., 'Artificial insemination: the attitude of patients in Norway', *Fert. & Ster.* (1951), 2, pp. 415–29.

27. Law of 21 April 1978, art. 33.

28. Law of 21 April 1977.

29. See Chapter 8.

30. (Israel) Rules Concerning the Administration of Sperm Banks and Directives for the Performance of Artificial Insemination 1979; (Switzerland) Guidelines on Medical Ethics Concerning Artificial Insemination (17 November 1981).

31. Krause, *Illegitimacy*, *passim*.

32. Jacob, op. cit., pp. 179–90; Holder, op. cit., pp. 225–38.

33. *Canterbury v. Spence* 464 F. 2d.772 (1972).

34. *Sidaway v. Bethlem Royal Hospital* [1985] 1 All ER 643 (HL).
35. *Bolam v. Friern Hospital Management Committee* [1957] 2 All ER 118; *Chatterton v. Gerson* [1981] 1 All ER 257; *Sidaway v. Board of Governors of the Bethlem Royal Hospital*, op. cit.
36. Holder, op. cit., pp. 230–4.
37. David, G. and Lausac, J., 'The organisation of the centers for the study and preservation of sperm in France', in David and Price, pp. 15–26.
38. Kritchevsky, B., 'The unmarried woman's right to artificial insemination: a call for expanded definition of family', *Harvard Women's Law Journal* (1981), 4, pp. 1–42, at 17–18.
39. Art. 16(1).
40. Art. 12.
41. Kritchevsky, op. cit., pp. 26–40.
42. 405 US 438 (1972).
43. Harris, L. E., 'Artificial insemination and surrogate motherhood', *Williamette LR* (1981), 17, pp. 913–34, at 934.
44. s.24(1).
45. s.3; for a fuller discussion see McLean, S., 'The right to reproduce' in Campbell, T., Goldberg, D., McLean, S. and Mullar, T., *Human Rights: from rhetoric to reality* (Blackwell, 1986), pp. 99–122.

Chapter 12

1. Leach, W. B., 'Perpetuities in the atomic age: the sperm bank and the fertile decedent', *ABAJ* (1962), 48, pp. 942–4, at 943. In 1971 it was reported in the *Wall Street Journal* that E. T. Tyler had announced to the American Medical Association that some males, prior to vasectomy, had deposited their semen as insurance (24 June, p. 16).
2. Sherman, J. K., 'Historical synopsis of human semen cryobanking' in David and Price, pp. 95–105, at 99.
3. *The Times*, 11 July, p. 3. See also Cusine, D. J., 'Artificial insemination with the husband's semen after death', *J. Med. Eth.* (1977), 3, pp. 163–5.
4. *The Times*, 11 July 1984.
5. ibid., 30 July 1985.
6. e.g. Human Tissue Act 1961 (UK); The Human Tissue Gift Act of Ontario (So. 1971), vol.2. c.83. Anatomical Donations and Post Mortem Examination Act 24 1970 (South Africa).
7. *Byers v. Byers*, 618 P. 2d. 930 (1980).
8. Law Reform (Miscellaneous Provisions) Act 1949.
9. Leach, op. cit., p. 942.
10. Sappideen, C., 'Life after death – sperm banks, wills and perpetuities', *Aus. LJ* (1979), 53, pp. 311–19; Cusine, D. J., 'Artificial insemination with the husband's semen after death', *J. Med. Eth.* (1977), 3, pp. 163–5.
11. There have been a number of proposals for dealing with the point, e.g. Thies, W. D., 'A look to the future: property rights and the posthumously conceived child', *Trusts and Estates* (1971), 110, pp. 922–3, 960. Some legislatures have rules on perpetuities which would deal with the point. See Sappideen, op. cit., p. 316.
12. Quinlivan, W. L. G. and Sullivan, M., 'The immunologic effects of husband's semen on donor spermatozoa during mixed insemination', *Fert. & Ster.* (1977), 24, pp. 448ff; Curie-Cohen *et al.*, 'Current practice of artificial insemination by donor in the United States', *NEJM* (1979), 300, pp. 585–90, at 587; Newton, J. R., RCOG (AI), p. 55.

13. Friedman, S., 'Artificial insemination with donor semen mixed with semen of the infertile husband', *Fert. & Ster.* (1980), 33, pp. 125–8.

Chapter 13

1. *Report of RCOG Ethics Committee on In Vitro Fertilisation and Embryo Replacement or Transfer*, March 1983, para. 5.3.
2. Warnock Report, para. 6.6.
3. *The Times*, 4 July 1986.
4. Edwards, R. G. and Steptoe, P. C., *A Matter of Life*. London, Hutchinson, 1980. The parents of Louise Brown published their account in Brown, L., Brown, J. and Freeman, S., *Our Miracle called Louise*. London, Paddington Press, 1979.
5. *Sunday Times*, 26 April 1986.
6. In 1978 it was reported that a woman had had a Fallopian tube transplant from her sister. This was done at a London hospital. *The Times*, 2 September 1978; see also Cohen, B. M., 'Current status of Fallopian tube transplantation', *Hosp. Practice* (1978), 13, pp. 87–94.
7. By April 1984 just over 200 children had been born as the result of IVF carried out by Steptoe and Edwards at their private clinic at Bourne Hall, Cambridge. There have been other births resulting from IVF done at other centres. Paper given by Mr Steptoe at BMA Scientific Meeting, Cambridge, April 1984.
8. Britain's first IVF triplets were born in London on 21 January 1984, and quadruplets in May 1984, also in London. Triplets were also born in Australia in January 1984.
9. This took place in Australia on 28 March 1984.
10. *Chatterton v. Gerson* [1981], 1 All ER 257.
11. *Nature* (1983), pp. 303, 336.
12. *Royal Commission on Civil Liability and Compensation for Personal Injury* (1978). Cmnd 7054, paras 1414–87 (UK); III, paras 134–7 (Canada); paras 766–9 (Australia); paras 436–7 (France); Prosser, W. L., *Handbook of the Law of Torts*, 6th edn (St Paul, Minn., West Pub., 1976), s. 55.
13. e.g. *Bonboest v. Katz*, 65F. Supp. 138 (DDC) (1946).
14. *Sylvia v. Gobeille* 220 A. 2d. 222 (1966).
15. *Zepeda v. Zepeda* 41 I11. App. 2d. 240 (1963).
16. *Williams v. State* 18 NY 2d. 481 (1966).
17. *Curlender v. Bio Science Laboratories* 106 Cal. App. 3d. 811 (1980).
18. *McKay v. Essex Area Health Authority* [1982] 2 All ER 771.
19. *Gleitman v. Cosgrove* 49 N.J. 22; 227 A 2d. (1967).
20. A claim by the parents was made in *McKay v. Essex*, op. cit., and was not ruled to be incompetent.
21. *Del Zio v. Manhattan's Columbia Presbyterian Medical Center* no. 74–3588 (SDNY) 1978.
22. e.g. *Thake v. Maurice* [1986] 1 All ER 497.
23. Edwards, R. G. and Steptoe, P. C., 'Current status of in vitro fertilisation and implantation of human embryos', *Lancet* (1983), 11, pp. 1265–9; Muasher, S. J. *et al.*, 'Benefits and risks of multiple transfer with in vitro fertilisation', ibid. (1984), II, p. 570.
24. *Report of Voluntary Licensing Authority for Human In Vitro Fertilisation and Embryology*. See *The Times*, 24 April 1986.
25. Scott, R., *The Body as Property* (London, Allen Lane, 1981), pp. 27–8.
26. ibid., pp. 189–93.

27. *Draft Recommendation on Artificial Insemination of Human Beings*, art. 6, and Explanatory Note 24. This is repeated in the Draft Recommendation on Human Artificial Procreation which was approved in April 1987.
28. Edwards, R. G., 'The current clinical and ethical situation of human conception in vitro' in Carter, C. O., ed., *Developments in Human Reproduction and their Eugenic, Ethical Implications* (London, Academic Press, pp. 102–3.
29. 'In vitro fertilisation: morality and public policy', evidence submitted to the Warnock Committee by the Catholic Bishops' Joint Committee on Bioethical Issues, para. 9.
30. Dunstan, G. R., 'The moral status of the human embryo: a tradition recalled', *J. Med. Eth.* (1984), 10, pp. 38–45.
31. Mahoney, J., *Bioethics and Belief* (London, Sheed & Ward, 1984), ch. 3.
32. *Brooks v. South Broward Hospital District* 325 So. 2d 479 (Fed. Dist. CA). 1975.
33. *The Use of Foetuses and Foetal Material for Research* (Peel Report) (London, HMSO, 1972), para. 42.
34. *Roe v. Wade* 410 US 113, at 160 (1973).
35. *Planned Parenthood of Central Missouri v. Danforth* 428 US 52 (1976); *Paton v. British Pregnancy Advisory Service Trustees* [1978] 2 *All ER*, 987. The case went to the European Court of Human Rights which rejected Mr Paton's contentions, (1980) 3 EHRR 408.
36. HC Deb. (11 May 1983), vol. 42, cols 238–9.
37. Dunstan, op. cit., n. 24.
38. HC Deb. vol. 28, cols 329–30 (written answer).
39. *Human Fertilisation and Embryology*. London, Royal Society, 1983.
40. *Research Related to Human Fertilisation and Embryology*. London, MRC, 1982; also *BMJ*, 285, p. 1480.
41. *Report of the RCOG Ethics Committee on In Vitro Fertilisation and Embryo Replacement or Transfer*.
42. 'Interim report on human in vitro fertilisation and embryo replacement and transfer', *BMJ* (1983), 286, pp. 1594–5.
43. *In Vitro Fertilisation: morality and public policy*. Abbots Langley, Catholic Information Services, 1983.
44. ibid., para. 11.
45. ibid., para. 9.
46. Report of USA Ethics Advisory Board (May 1979), p. 101.
47. For a full account of activities in the USA see Abramovitch, S., 'A stalemate on test-tube baby research', *Hastings Center Report* (1984), 14, no. 1, pp. 5–9.
48. Australian Law Reform Commission, 7, 18.
49. Artificial Conception Act 1984, which came into force on 1 August (NSW): Infertility Medical Procedures Act 1984 (Victoria). As at 30 September 1986, very little of the Act is in force.
50. Cusine, D. J., 'Some legal implications of embryo transfer', *Lancet* (1979), 2, pp. 407–8.
51. RCOG: *Report of the RCOG Ethics Committee on In Vitro Fertilisation and Embryo Replacement or Transfer*. London, 1983; BMA, Interim Report, op. cit., *BMJ* (1983), 286, 1594–5.

CHAPTER 14

1. Mason, J. K. and McCall-Smith, R. A., *Law and Medical Ethics* (London, Butterworths, 1983), p. 45.
2. Snowden, Mitchell and Snowden, pp. 32–8.
3. Gen. 16:1–3; 30:1–6.

4. Hearings before the Sub-Committee on Children and Youth of the Committee on Labor and Public Welfare. 94th Congress, 1st Session, *Baby Sitting*, 28 and 29 April 1975.

5. ibid., pp. 4–5.

6. McTaggart, L., 'How I sold – and almost bought a baby', *Sunday New York News Magazine*, 13 April 1975.

7. Areen, p. 1158.

8. *Sosna v Iowa* 419 US 393 (1975).

9. *Smith v. Organisation of Foster Families* 431 US 291 (1977).

10. *Loving v. Virginia* 388 US 1 (1967).

11. *Planned Parenthood of Missouri v. Danforth* 428 US 52 (1976).

12. *Griswold v. Connecticut* 318 US 479 (1965).

13. *Roe v. Wade* 410 US 113 (1973).

14. Goldstein, J., Freud A. and Solnit, A. J., *Beyond the Best Interests of the Child* (London, Burnett Books, 1980), pp. 16–17.

15. *Doe v. Kelley* 106 Mich. 169 (1981).

16. *Scotsman*, 4 March 1986.

17. Adoption (Scotland) Act 1978 s.51; Adoption Act 1976 s.57 (E & W).

18. Clark, p. 340.

19. *Cal. Penal Code* s.273.

20. *Mich. Comp.* Law. Ann s.710.5.

21. Ill. Rev. Stat. ch. 4 s.12–1; 12–5.

22. NJ Stat. Ann. s.2A 96–97.

23. ss 1181–3.

24. Brock, J., 'California's adoption law and programs', *Hastings Law Journal* (1955), 6, pp. 261–350; note 'Black market adoptions', *Cath. Lawyer* (1976), 22, pp. 48ff.

25. *Hooks v. Bridgewater* 229 SW 1114 (1921).

26. *Willey v. Lawton* 132 NE 2d. 34 (1956).

27. e.g. *Chapsky v. Wood* 26 Kan. 650 (1881). per Justice Brewer; Children Act 1975 s. 3 (UK).

28. *People ex rel Scarpetta v. Spence Chaplin Adoption Service* 269 NE 2d. 787 (1971). In the UK the child stays with the intended adopters for a trial period of at least 13 weeks, Adoption Act 1976 s.13; Adoption (Scotland) Act 1978 s.13.

29. *US v. Enmous* 410 US 396, 411 (1973) Justice Stewart; *IRC v. Hinchy* [1960] AC 748.

30. *Webster v. Rotary Electric Steel Co* 321 Mich. 526; (1948) *Nokes v. Doncaster Amalgamated Collieries* [1940] AC 1014.

31. *Re an adoption application (surrogacy)* [1987] 2 All ER. 806

32. s. 50(1).

33. s. 50(3).

34. Cotton, K. and Winn, D., *Baby Cotton: for love and money*. (London, Dorling Kindersley, 1985.)

35. *The Times*, 2 July 1986.

36. Births and Deaths Registration Act 1953 s.1; Registration of Births, Deaths and Marriages (Scotland) Act 1965 s.14.

37. *Chitty on Contracts*, 25th edn (London, Sweet & Maxwell, 1983), ch. 3; Corbin, Al, *Contracts* (St Paul, Minn., West Publishing, 1951), s. 111.

38. Chitty, op. cit., para. 158; Corbin, op. cit., ss 122, 131.

39. e.g. Scots law, see Gloag, W. M., *The Law of Contract*, 2nd edn (Edinburgh, Green, 1929), p. 48.

40. Chitty, op. cit., para. 41; Corbin, op. cit., s.9; Gloag, op. cit., pp. 16–27.

41. Chitty, op. cit., paras 1033–42; Corbin, op. cit., s.1374ff ; Gloag, op. cit., pp. 550–2.

42. (1968), 186 Kan. 311.
43. ibid., 320.
44. ibid., 324.
45. ibid., 325.
46. (1975), 519 F 2d. 187.
47. ibid., 190.
48. ibid., 189.
49. 6. Fam. L. Rep. (BNA) 3011; 106 Mich. App. 169; 307 NW 2d 38 (1981).
50. *Surrogate Parenting Assoc. Inc. v. Kentucky* 12 Fam. L. Rep (BNA) 1207 (1986).
51. 217 N.J. Super. 313; 525 A 2d 1128 (1987).
52. Note 'Moppets on the market: the problem of unregulated adoptions', *Yale Law Journal* (1950), 59, pp. 715ff.
53. e.g. Australia, Canada.
54. Adoption (Scotland) Act 1978 s.11; Adoption Act 1976 s.11.
55. e.g. Adoption (Scotland) Act 1978 s.11; Adoption Act 1976 s.11.
56. e.g. Adoption (Scotland) Act 1978 s.15; Adoption Act 1976 s.15.
57. *Adoption of H* 69 Misc. 2d. 304 (1972).
58. e.g. 'Woman having baby for transsexual sister', *The Times*, 17 January 1981.
59. *Guardian*, 9 March 1986.
60. Chitty, op. cit., para. 1705; MacNeil, I. R., *Contracts* (New York, Foundation Press, 1978), pp. 96–8.
61. Chitty, op. cit., paras 1401–3; Corbin, op. cit., paras 1355ff; Gloag, op. cit., pp. 337ff.
62. Chitty, op. cit., para. 1763; Corbin, op. cit., para. 993.
63. Chitty, op. cit., para. 1761; Corbin, op. cit., para. 1136; Gloag, op. cit., p. 655.
64. *Stewart v. Rudner*, 84 NYS 2d 816 (1971).
65. Chitty, op. cit., para. 1771; Corbin, op. cit., paras 1204–9, Gloag, op. cit., p. 657.
66. Adoption (Scotland) Act 1978 s.13(1); Adoption Act 1976 s.13 (UK); *People ex rel Scarpetta v. Spence Chaplin Adoption Service* 28 NYS 2d. 185 (1971) (USA).
67. Cretney, ch. 12; Krause, *Family Law*, ch. 17.
68. *A v. C* (1978), 6 *Family Law* 170.
69. e.g. Adoption (Scotland) Act 1978 s.15; Adoption Act 1976 s.15 (E & W); Krause, *Family Law*, p. 1105 (USA).
70. Titmus, R., *The Gift Relationship* (New York, Pantheon, 1971), *passim*.
71. *The Times*, 2 July 1986.
72. Council for Science and Society, *Human Procreation: ethical aspects of the new techniques* (Oxford University Press 1984), pp. 69–70.
73. Brahams, D., 'Warnock Report', *Lancet* (1984), 1, pp. 238–9.

Chapter 15

1. Warnock, para. 9.11.
2. Snowden, Mitchell and Snowden, p. 161.
3. ibid., p. 174.

Chapter 16

1. 28 HL Deb., 6th ser. 1, col. 329 (23 July 1982).
2. The Report is hereafter referred to as Warnock.
3. 'Artificial insemination', 128 HL Deb., 5th ser., cols 816–6 (28 July 1943);

Human Artificial Insemination. Report of the Archbishop of Canterbury's Commission. London, SPCK, 1948; 'Problems of legitimacy and artificial insemination' 161 HL Deb., 5th ser., cols 386–429 (16 March 1949); 'Artificial insemination of married women', 207 HL Deb., 5th ser., cols 926–1016 (26 February 1958); *Report of the Departmental Committee on Human Artificial Insemination*. Cmnd 1105. HMSO, 1960; 'Human artificial insemination', *BMJ* (1973), 2, Supp. (7 April), pp. 3–5.

4. Warnock, para. 1.2.
5. ibid., para. 1.6.
6. ibid., paras 1.9–1.10.
7. ibid., para. 1.9.
8. ibid., chs 4–8.
9. ibid., paras 3.4, 9.3.
10. ibid., para. 2.16.
11. *Report of the RCOG Working Party on Further Specialisations within Obstetrics and Gynaecology*. London, RCOG, 1982.
12. Warnock, para. 2.17.
13. ibid., para. 3.14.
14. ibid., para. 3.5.
15. ibid., para. 3.2.
16. ibid.
17. ibid., para. 4.26.
18. ibid., para. 6.6.
19. ibid., para. 4.27.
20. David, G. and Lansac, J., 'The organisation of centers for the study and preservation of semen in France' in David and Price, pp. 15–25, at 20.
21. *Draft Recommendation of Artificial Insemination of Human Beings* (1979), art. 6.
22. Warnock, paras 13.3–13.4.
23. *The Times*, 23 January 1985.
24. ibid., 21 January 1986.
25. Warnock, para. 4.5.
26. ibid., para. 4.16.
27. ibid., para. 4.17.
28. Feversham Report, Memorandum of Dissent, para. 14.
29. *Family Law: illegitimacy* (London, HMSO, 1982), paras 12.9–12.11.
30. Warnock, para. 4.24.
31. ibid., para. 4.22.
32. ibid., para. 4.25.
33. ibid., para. 4.21.
34. ibid., para. 6.1.
35. ibid., para. 6.6.
36. ibid., para. 6.7.
37. ibid., para. 6.8.
38. ibid., para. 5.10.
39. ibid., para. 5.11.
40. Trounson, A. *et al.*, 'Pregnancy established in an infertile patient after transfer of a donated embryo fertilised in vitro', *BMJ* (1983), 286, pp. 835–8.
41. Warnock, para. 7.6.
42. ibid., para. 7.7.
43. ibid., para. 7.1.
44. ibid., para. 7.5.
45. *The Times*, 7 February 1984; Annas, G. J., 'Surrogate embryo transfer: the perils of parenting', *Hastings Center Report* (1984), 11, no. 3, pp. 25–6.
46. Warnock, para. 8.1.

47. ibid., para. 8.2.
48. ibid., paras 8.3–8.4.
49. ibid., para. 8.2.
50. *A v. C* (1978), 6 *Fam. Law* 170; see ch. 17 for details.
51. Cusine, D. J., 'Womb-leasing: some legal implications', *New L.J.* (1978), 128, pp. 824–6.
52. Warnock, para. 8.7.
53. ibid., para. 8.6.
54. ibid., para. 8.9.
55. ibid., para. 8.13.
56. ibid., para. 8.14.
57. ibid.
58. ibid., para. 8.15.
59. ibid., para. 8.16.
60. ibid., paras 8.10–8.12.
61. ibid., para. 8.17.
62. ibid., para. 8.18.
63. Editorial, *Lancet* (1984), 1, pp. 202–4.
64. 'Artificial fertilisation made natural', *Nature* (1984), 301, p. 269.
65. Warnock, Expression of Dissent A, paras 1–9. One of the dissenters, David Davies, expanded on his reasons for dissenting in *The Times*, 19 July 1984.
66. Warnock, para. 9.3.
67. ibid., para. 9.12.
68. ibid., para. 9.11.
69. Swinbanks, D., 'Gender selection sparks row', *Nature* (1986), 321, p. 720.
70. Warnock, para. 10.9.
71. ibid., para. 10.2.
72. ibid., para. 10.3.
73. ibid., para. 10.8.
74. ibid., para. 10.8.
75. ibid., para. 10.10.
76. Statement on In Vitro Fertilisation and Embryo Transfer, 3 September 1982.
77. Warnock, para. 10.10.
78. ibid., paras 10.12–10.13.
79. ibid., para. 10.12.
80. ibid.
81. *The Times*, 18 June 1984. Despite requests by some Australian women to have the embryos implanted in them, they remained frozen as at 29 August 1985. See ed. n. in Smith, G. P., II, 'Australia's frozen orphan embryos: a medical, legal and ethical dilemma', *J. Fam. Law* (1985), 24, pp. 27–41, at 41.
82. Warnock, para. 10.13.
83. ibid., para. 10.11.
84. ibid., para. 13.13.
85. ibid., para. 10.14.
86. ibid., para. 10.15.
87. Expressions of Dissent B and C, pp. 90–4.
88. *The Times*, 21, 23, 25, 31 July 1984.
89. Warnock, para. 11.10.
90. See Edwards, R. and Steptoe, P., *A Matter of Life* (London, Hutchinson, 1980), ch. 13.
91. Warnock, para. 11.22.
92. ibid., paras 11.11–11.12.
93. ibid., para. 11.13.
94. ibid., para. 11.14.

95. Expression of Dissent B, pp. 90–3, para. 3.
96. ibid., para. 5.
97. See Kuhse, H. and Singer, P., 'The moral status of the embryo' in Walters and Singer, pp. 57–63, esp. pp. 61–3.
98. See Glover, J., *Causing Death and Saving Lives* (Harmondsworth, Penguin, 1977), esp. chs 6 and 15; Rachels, J., 'Active and passive euthanasia', *NEJM* (1975), 292, pp. 78–80.
99. Warnock, para. 11.15.
100. Dunstan, G. R., 'The moral status of the human embryo: a tradition recalled', *J. Med. Eth.* (1984), 10, no. 1, pp. 38–44. For a contrary view in the same issue see Iglesias, T., 'In vitro fertilisation: the major issues', pp. 32–7.
101. Warnock, paras. 11.15–11.16.
102. ibid., para. 11.18 and n. 2.
103. *The Use of Foetuses and Foetal Material for Research* Peel Report. London, HMSO, 1972.
104. Warnock, para. 11.18 n.2.
105. ibid., para. 11.22.
106. 'Interim report on human *in vitro* fertilisation and embryo replacement and transfer', *BMJ* (1983), 286, pp. 1594–5 (BMA); 'Research related to human fertilisation and embryology'. London, MRC, 1982.
107. Ethics Advisory Board, *Health Education and Welfare Support of Research involving Human In Vitro Fertilisation and Embryo Transfer* (Washington, DC, 1979), p. 107.
108. Warnock, para. 11.5.
109. ibid., para. 11.20.
110. *Human Fertilisation and Embryology* (London, Royal Society, 1983), para. 13.
111. *Report of the RCOG Ethics Committee on In Vitro Fertilisation and Embryo Replacement or Transfer* (London, RCOG, 1983), para. 13.8.
112. 'Backing sought to grow embryos for up to thirty days', *Guardian*, 16 April 1984.
113. Warnock, para. 11.24.
114. Expression of dissent C, p. 94.
115. Warnock, paras 11.25–11.27.
116. ibid., para. 11.28.
117. ibid., para. 11.30.
118. ibid., ch. 12.
119. ibid., para. 12.1.
120. ibid., paras 12.2–12.16.
121. ibid., paras 12.15–12.16.
122. ibid., para. 9.3.
123. ibid., paras 12.2–12.3.
124. Yanigamachi, R. *et al.*, 'The use of zona-free animal ova as a test system for the assessment of the fertilisation capacity of human spermatozoa', *Biological Reproduction* (1976), 15, pp. 471ff.
125. Warnock, para. 12.3.
126. ibid., para. 12.5–12.6.
127. ibid., paras 12.7–12.8.
128. ibid., para. 12.9.
129. Heape, W., 'Preliminary note on the transplantation and growth of mammalian ova within a uterine foster mother', *Proc. Royal Society (B. Biological Sciences)* (1890), 48, pp. 457–8; Rowson, L. E. A. and Morr, R. M., 'Non-surgical transfer of cow eggs', *J. Reprod. & Fert.* (1966), 11, pp. 311–12.
130. Warnock, para. 12.10.
131. Cherfas, J. and Gribbin, J., *The Redundant Male*. London, Bodley Head, 1984.

132. Warnock, para. 12.11.
133. Gurdon, J. B. and Laskey, R. A., 'The transplantation of nuclei from single cultured cells', *J. Embryology and Experimental Morphology* (1970), 24, pp. 227–48.
134. 'Human embryo banks proposed', *The Times*, 28 January 1982.
135. David Rorvik, *In his Image: the cloning of a man*. New York, Lippincott, 1978.
136. e.g. Haldane, J. B. S., 'Biological possibilities in the next 10 000 years' in Wolstenholme, G., ed., *Man and his future*. London, Churchill, 1963; Ledenburg, J., 'Experimental genetics and human evolution', *Bulletin of the Atomic Scientists* (1966), pp. 4–11.
137. Warnock, paras. 12.12–12.13.
138. ibid., para. 12.13.
139. Edwards, R. G., 'What now for test-tube babies?', *New Scientist* (1982), 93, pp. 312–16, at 313.
140. Warnock, para. 12.14.
141. Edwards, R. G., 'The Galton Lecture 1982; id. the current clinical and ethical situation of human conception *in vitro*' in Carter, C. O., ed., *Developments in Human Reproduction and their Eugenic, Ethical Implications* (London, Academic Press, 1983), pp. 53–116, at 105–9.
142. Warnock, para. 1.7.
143. ibid., para. 13.1.
144. ibid., Foreword, para. 5.
145. ibid., para. 13.1.
146. ibid., para. 13.2.
147. ibid.
148. ibid., para. 13.3.
149. ibid., para. 13.4.
150. ibid., para. 13.5.
151. ibid., para. 13.6.
152. Similar provisions exist in relation to anatomy and other subjects, e.g. Anatomy Act 1984.

Chapter 17

1. *The Times*; *Guardian*; *Daily Telegraph*, 21 July 1984.
2. e.g. correspondence, 23, 25, 27, 31 July; 7, 8, 9 August; 26 November; 28 December 1984; 8, 14 January 1985.
3. Press releases, 18 July 1984.
4. HC Deb., vol. 73, col. 685 (15 February 1985).
5. 'Human fertilisation: Warnock Report', HL Deb., vol. 456, cols 535–93 (31 October 1984).
6. 'Human fertilisation and embryology (Warnock Report)', HC Deb., vol. 68, cols 528–90 (28 November 1984).
7. *Human Fertilisation and Embryology: A Framework for Legislation*, Department of Health and Social Security, November 1987 cm 259.
8. e.g. Lord Meston, HL Deb., vol. 456, col. 583; Lord Prys-Davies, ibid., col. 586.
9. e.g. Marquess of Reading, ibid., col. 537; Lord Coleraine, ibid., col. 546; Lord Rawlinson of Ewell, ibid., cols 555–6; Marquess of Lothian, ibid., col. 566; Lady Saltoun, ibid., col. 563; Lord Ashbourne, ibid., col. 568; Lord Tranmire, ibid., col. 574; Lord Longford, ibid., col. 575.
10. Marquess of Reading, ibid., col. 536; Lord Denning, ibid., col. 542; Lord Rawlinson of Ewell, ibid., col. 556; Earl of Halsbury, ibid., col. 558.

11. Lord Coleraine, ibid., col. 546; Bishop of Norwich, ibid., col. 553; Earl of Halsbury, ibid., col. 558; Lady Saltoun, ibid., col. 563; Lord Milverton, ibid., col. 579.
12. Marquess of Reading, ibid., col. 535; Lord Denning, ibid., col. 542; Lord Rawlinson of Ewell, ibid., col. 555; Lord Robertson of Oakbridge, ibid., col. 567; Lord Ashbourne, ibid., col. 570.
13. ibid., col. 542.
14. ibid., col. 539.
15. ibid., col. 556.
16. ibid., col. 580.
17. ibid., cols 546–9.
18. ibid., cols 584–7.
19. ibid., cols 587–93.
20. ibid., col. 548.
21. ibid.
22. ibid., col. 585.
23. ibid., col. 586.
24. ibid., col. 577.
25. ibid., col. 590.
26. HC Deb., vol. 73, cols 528–34.
27. Edwards, R. G., 'Fertilisation of human eggs in vitro: morals, ethics and the law', Quar. Rev. Biology (1974), 49, pp. 3ff.
28. e.g. Sunday Times, 4 June 1978.
29. e.g. Harry Greenway, HC Deb., vol. 73, col. 531; Revd Ian Paisley, ibid., col. 554; Sir Hugh Rossi, ibid., col. 562; John Hume, ibid., col. 569; W. Benyon, ibid., col. 582; Peter Bruinvels, ibid., col. 582.
30. ibid., cols 536–8.
31. ibid., cols 543–50.
32. e.g. Peter Bruinvels.
33. HC Deb., vol. 73, cols 587–8.
34. The Times, 21 July 1984.
35. 'Human reproduction: regulated progress or damned interference', Lancet (1984), 2, pp. 202–4.
36. 'Artificial fertilisation made natural', Nature (1984), 310, p. 269.
37. The Times, 3 August 1984.
38. A v. C [1978], 6 Fam. Law. 170.
39. In Re Baby M, 217 N.J. Super. 313; 525A 2d 1128 (1987).
40. Cotton, K. and Winn, D., Baby Cotton: for love and money. London, Dorling Kindersley, 1985.
41. Children and Young Persons Act 1969, s. 1.
42. The Times, 7 January 1985.
43. Sunday Times, 13 January 1985.
44. Surrogacy Arrangements Act 1985, s. 2.
45. paras 73–74.
46. Scotsman, 4 March 1986.
47. The Times, 2 July 1986.
48. Guardian, 9 March 1986.
49. The Times, 26 June 1986.
50. ibid., 26 June 1985.
51. HC Deb., vol. 73, col. 684.
52. The Times, 26 November 1984.
53. ibid., 23 January 1985.
54. In April 1986 and April 1987.

55. *Human Fertilisation and Embryology: A Framework for Legislation, Department of Health and Social Security, Nov. 1987 Cm* 259 paras 8–11.
56. *Legislation on Human Infertility Services and Embryo Research*: A Consultation Paper, Department of Health and Social Security, June 1986, Cm. 46.
57. paras. 28–30.
58. paras. 8–12, 15.
59. para. 27.
60. paras. 36–42.
61. paras. 43–58.
62. paras. 59–60.
63. paras. 72–75.
64. Family Law Reform Act 1987 s.27.
65. para. 89.
66. para.
67. para. 86.
68. Royal Commission on Family and Children's Law, 9th Report, *Artificial Insemination*. 1975.
69. Alberta Institute of Law Research and Reform, *Report on Status of Children*, Report no. 20. 1976.
70. Law Reform Commission of Saskatchewan, *Tentative Proposals for a Human Artificial Insemination Act*. 1981.
71. Quebec Civil Code Act, 586; Children's Act 1984.
72. *Report on Human Artificial Reproduction and Related Matters*. Ontario Law Commission, 1985. (Ontario Report)
73. ibid., Recommendations 3–18.
74. ibid., 19–21.
75. ibid., 26–7.
76. ibid., 29–33.
77. ibid., 34–66.
78. Ethics Advisory Board, *New Support of Research Involving Human In Vitro Fertilisation and Embryo Transfer* (1979), pp. 108–12.
79. Ill. Stat. Ann., ch. 38, 81–26(9) (Supp. 1983/84).
80. *Smith v. Fahner*.
81. Ontario Report, op. cit., 2, pp. 382–83.
82. ibid., p. 381.
83. For the background, see the New South Wales Report *infra* ch. 1.
84. New South Wales – Discussion Paper November 1984; Report July 1986; Queensland – Report 1984; South Australia – Report of Working Party January 1984; Report of Select Committee April 1987; Tasmania – Report June 1985; Victoria – Committee to Consider the Social, Ethical and Legal Issues arising from In Vitro Fertilization. (i) Interim Report (1982); (ii) Report on Donor Gametes (1983); Report on the Disposition of Embryos Produced by In Vitro Fertilization (1984); Western Australia – Interim Report August 1984; Report September 1986.
85. see fn. 84.
86. see 1984 Report.
87. *The Times*, 25 October 1984.
88. L. Waller 'In Australia, The Debate Moves to Embryo Experimentation', *Hastings Center Report*, June 1987, pp. 21–22.
89. see fn. 84.
90. see fn. 84.
91. New South Wales Law Reform Commission: *Surrogate Motherhood: Australian Public Opinion* May 1987.
92. see fn. 84.

93. see fn. 84.
94. Tasmania: Status of Children Amendment Act 1985; Western Australia: Artificial Conception Act 1985; Capital Territory: Artificial Conception Ordinance 1985; Northern Territory: Status of Children Amendment Act 1985
95. *Human Embryo Experimentation in Australia.* 1986.
96. This information is derived from a paper presented by M. Byk at the United Kingdom Comparative Law Colloquium, Cambridge, August 1987.
97. *Instruction on Respect for Human Life in its Origins and on the Dignity of Procreation.* March 1987. For full text, see *The New York Times*, 11 March 1987, p. 10.
98. *The Times*, 11 October 1982.

Bibliography

Abramovitch, S. 'A stalemate on test-tube baby research', *Hastings Center Report* (1984), 14, no. 1.

Alberta Institute of Law Research, *Status of Children*, Report no. 20 (1976).

Annas, G. J., 'Artificial insemination: beyond the best interests of the donor', *Hastings Center Report* (1979), 9, no. 4.

Annas, G. J., 'Surrogate embryo transfer: the perils of parenting', *Hastings Center Report* (1984), 11, no. 3.

Areen, J., *Cases and Materials on Family Law*. New York, Foundation Press, 1978.

'Artificial fertilisation made natural', *Nature* (1984), 301.

Ashbourne, Ld, in HL Debates, vol. 456, cols 568, 570.

'Australia's wonder baby', *The Times*, 13 January 1984.

'Backing sought to grow embryos for up to thirty days', *Guardian*, 16 April 1984.

Barkay, J. and Zuckerman, H., 'AID and sperm bank development in Israel' in David and Price.

Bartholomew, G. P., 'Legal aspects of artificial insemination', *Mod. Law Rev.* (1958), 21.

Barton, E., in *Medical World*.

Barton, M., Walker, K. and Wiesner, B. P., 'Artificial insemination', *BMJ* (1945), 1.

Behrman, S. J., 'Artificial insemination' in Behrman and Kistner.

Behrman, S. J. and Kistner, R. W., 'A rational approach to the evaluation of infertility' in Behrman and Kistner.

Behrman and Kistner, *Progress in Infertility*, 2nd edn. Boston, Little, Brown, 1975.

Benyon, W., in HC Debates, vol. 73, col. 582.

'Black market adoptions', *Cath. Lawyer* (1976), 22.

Blackstone, W., *Commentaries on the Laws of England*, ed. Kerr, R. M. (London, Murray, 1862), I.

BMA Panel, 'Report of the British Medical Association p n 1 on human artificial insemination', *BMJ* (1973), 2, supp. (7 April).

Brahams, D., 'Warnock Report', *Lancet* (1984), 1.

Bremond, A. *et al.*, 'Evaluation of female fertility before AID' in David and Price.

Brock, J., 'California's adoption law and programs', *Hastings Law Journal* (1955), 6.

Bromley, P. M., *Family Law*, 6th edn. London, Butterworths, 1981.

Brown, L., Brown, J. and Freeman, S., *Our Miracle called Louise*, London, Paddington Press, 1979.

Bruinvels, Peter, in HC Debates, vol. 73, col. 582.

Caldwell, J. H., 'Babies by scientific selection', *Scientific American* (1934), 150.

Cal. Penal Code.

Campana, A. *et al.*, 'Present status of AID and sperm banks in Switzerland' in David and Price.

Campbell, T., Goldberg, D., McLean, S. and Mullar, T., *Human Rights: from rhetoric to reality*. Blackwell, 1986.

Carter, C. O., ed., *Developments in Human Reproduction and their Eugenic, Ethical Implications*. London, Academic Press, 1983.

Case Reports

  A. v. C. [1978], 6 Family Law 170.

  AB v. CD (1854) 14 D. 177.

  AB v. CD (1904), 7 F. 72.

  Adoption of H., 69 Misc. 2d. 304 (1972).

  Anon v. Anon, 41 Misc. 2d. 886; 246 NYS 2d. 835 (1964).

  Att. Gen. v. Mulholland [1963] 2 QB. 477.

  Baxter v. Baxter [1948] AC. 274.

  Bell v. Bell (1909) 75. 500.

  Bolam v. Friern Hospital Management Committee [1957] 2 A11 ER, 118.

  Bonboest v. Katz, 65 F. Supp. 138 (DDC) (1946).

  Bravery v. Bravery [1954] 1 WLR, 1169.

  Brooks v. South Broward Hospital District, 325 So. 2d. 479 (Fed. Dist. CA) (1975).

  Byers v. Byers, 618 P 2d. 930 (1980).

  Cackett v. Cackett [1950] P 253.

  Canterbury v. Spence, 464 F. 2d. 772 (1972).

  Carey v. Population Services International, 431 US. 678 (1977).

  Carter v. Inter Faith Hospital of Queens, 60 Misc. 2d. 733 (1969).

  Chapsky v. Wood, 26 Kan. 650 (1881).

  Chatterton v. Gerson and anr, [1981] 1 All ER, 257.

  Clarke v. Clarke [1943] 2 All ER, 540.

  Cowen v. Cowen [1946] P 36.

  Curlender v. Bio Science Laboratories, 106 Cal. App. 3d. 811 (1980).

  D. v. A. (1845) 1 Rob. Ecc. 279.

  Del Zio v. Manhattan's Columbia Presbyterian Medical Center (1978), no. 74–3588 (SDNY).

Doe v. Kelley, 106 Mich. 169 (1981).

Doornbos v. Doornbos (1954), Unreported 1945 no. 44–C–9307, Cir. Ct., Cook Co., Ill.

Dumer v. St Michael's Hospital, 69 Wisc. 2d. 233; 233 NW. 2d. 372, Sup. Ct., Wisc. (1978).

Eisenstadt v. Baird, 405 US 438 (1972).

Frontiero v. Richardson, 411 US 677 (1973).

G. v. G. 1961 SLT 324; SC 347.

Gillick v. West Norfolk and Wisbech Area Health Authority [1985] 3 All ER, 402 (HL).

Gleitman v. Cosgrove, 49 NJ 22; 227 A. 2d. (1967).

Grimes v. Grimes [1948] P 323.

Griswold v. Connecticut, 318 US 479 (1965).

Gursky v. Gursky (1963) 39 Misc. 2d. 1083; 242 NYS 2d. 406.

Hall v. Brooklands Auto-Racing Club [1933] 1 KB 205.

Hoch v. Hoch (1945), Unreported 1945, no. 44–C–9307, Cir. Ct., Cook Co., Ill.

Hooks v. Bridgewater, 229 SW 1114 (1921).

Hunter v. Hanley 1955, S.C 200.

Hyde v. Hyde (1866), LR, 1 P & D 130.

In re Adoption of Anonymous, 74 Misc. 2d. 99; 345 NYS 2d. 430, (1973).

In re Ann Carol S, NYLJ, (1974).

In re Shirk, 186 Kan. 311 (1968).

IRC v. Hinchy [1960] AC 748.

J. v. J. 1978 SLT 128.

Jimenez v. Weinberger, 417 US 628 (1974).

Levy v. Louisiana, 391 US 68 (1968).

Lovallo v. NJ State Register, 148 NJ Super. 302 (1977).

Loving v. Virginia, 388 US 1 (1967).

McGowan v. Maryland, 366 US 420 (1961).

McKay v. Essex Health Authority [1982], 2 All ER, 771.

MacLennan v. MacLennan 1958 SC 105; SLT 12.

Manbeck v. Manbeck, 339 Pa Super. 493; 489 A. 2d. 748.

Nokes v. Doncaster Amalgamated Collieries [1940] AC 1014.

Ohlsen v. Ohlsen, Sup. Ct., Cook Co., Ill. (1954).

Orford v. Orford (1921) 59 DLR, 251.

Paton v. British Pregnancy Advisory Service Trustees [1978], 2 All ER, 987.

People ex rel Abajian v. Dennett, 184 NYS 2d. 178; 15 Misc. 2d. 260 (1958).

People ex rel Scarpetta v. Spence Chaplin Adoption Service, 269 NE 2d. 787 (1971).

People v. Sorensen, 437 P. 2d. 495; 66 Cal. Rep. 285; 68 Cal. Rep. 7 (1968).

Perlmutter v. Beth David Hospital, 308 NY 100; 123 NE 2d. 792 (1954).

Pfizer Corporation v. Ministry of Health [1965], AC 512.

Planned Parenthood of Central Missouri v. Danforth (1976), 428 US 52.

Ravenis v. Detroit General Hospital, 63 Mich. App. 79; 234 NW 2d. 411 (1978).

Reed v. Reed, 404 US 71 (1971).

Reimche v. First National Bank of Nevada, 519 F. 2d. 187 (1975).

R.E.L. v. E.L. [1949] P 211.

Roberts v. Roberts (1971) VR 160.

Roe v. Wade, 410 US 113 (1973).

Russell v. Russell [1924] AC 687.

Sapsford v. Sapsford [1954] P 394.

Sidaway v. Bethlem Royal Hospital [1985] 1 *All ER*, 643 (HL).

Skinner v. Oklahoma, 316 US 535 (1942).

Slater v. Slater [1953] P 235.

Smith v. Fahner, no. 82, c4324 (Ill.) (1982).

Smith v. Organisation of Foster Families, 431 US 291 (1977).

Sosna v. Iowa, 419 US 393 (1975).

State v. Roberts, 169 Wisc. (1919).

Stewart v. Rudner, 84 NYS 2d. 816 (1971).

Strnad v. Strnad, 190 Misc. 786; 78 NYS 2d. 390 (1948).

Sylvia v. Gobeille, 220 A. 2d. 222 (1966).

Syrkowski v. Appleyard 122 Mich. App. 506; 333 NW 2d. 90 (1983).

T. v. M., 100 NJ Super. 530; 242 A. 2d. 670 (1968).

Thake v. Maurice [1986] 1 *All ER*, 497.

US v. Enmous, 410 US 396, 411 (1973).

V. v. R. (1979), (3) SA 1006.

Vigil v. Rice, 397 P. 2d. 719 (1964).

W. v. Official Solicitor [1972] AC 24.

Weber v. Aetna Casualty and Surety Co., 406 US 164 (1972).

Webster v. Rotary Electric Steel Co., 321 Mich. 526 (1948).

White v. White [1948] P 330.

Whitehouse v. Jordon [1981] 1 *All ER*, 267 (HL).

Willey v. Lawton, 132 NE 2d. 34 (1956).

Williams v. State, 18 NY 2d. 481 (1966).

Zepeda v. Zepeda, 41 Ill. App. 2d. 240 (1963).

Chamberlain, G. and Brown, J. C., 'Complication of laparoscopy' in *Gynaecological Laparoscopy*. Report of Working Party of the Confidential Inquiry into Gynaecological Laparoscopy. RCOG, 1978.

Chandler, H. S., 'A legislative approach to artificial insemination', *Cornell LR* (1968), 53.

Chappel, A., 'Artificial insemination', *J. American Medical Women's Assoc.* (1959), 14.

Cherfas, J. and Gribbin, J., *The Redundant Male.* London, Bodley Head, 1984.

Chester, R., 'Is there a relationship between childlessness and marriage breakdown?', *J. Biosocial Science* (1971), 4.

Children Conceived by Artificial Insemination. SOU, 1983.

Chitty on Contracts, 25th edn. London, Sweet & Maxwell, 1983.

The Church and the Law of Nullity of Marriage. London, SPCK, 1955.

Ciba Foundation, *Law and Ethics of AID and Embryo Transfer.* Symposium no. 17, n.s. Elsevier, Excerpta Medica, 1973.

Clark, H. H., *Cases and Problems on Domestic Relations*, 2nd edn. St Paul, Minn., West Pub., 1974.

Clerk, J. F. and Lindsell, W. H., The Law of Torts, 15th edn. London, Sweet & Maxwell, 1974.

Clive, E. M., *The Law of Husband and Wife in Scotland*, 2nd edn. Edinburgh, Green, 1982.

Clyde, Ld Pres., in *Hunter v. Hanley* (1955).

Cohen, B. M., 'Current status of Fallopian tube transplantation', *Hosp. Practice* (1978), 13.

Coleraine, Ld, in HL Debates, vol. 456, col. 546.

Consumers' Assoc., *Infertility.* London, 1969.

Corbin, A. L., *Contracts.* St Paul, Minn., West Pub., 1951.

Corpus Iuris Secundum. St Paul, Minn., West Pub., 1974.

Cotton, K. and Winn, D., *Baby Cotton: for love and money.* London, Dorling Kindersley, 1985.

Council for Science and Society, *Human Procreation: ethical aspects of the new techniques.* Oxford University Press, 1984.

Cretney, S. M., *Principles of Family Law*, 4th edn. London, Sweet & Maxwell, 1984.

Curie-Cohen, M. *et al.*, 'Current practice of artificial insemination by donor in the United States', *NEJM* (1979), 300.

Cusine, D. J., 'Some legal implications of embryo transfer', *Lancet* (1979), 2.

Cusine, D. J., 'Artificial insemination with the husband's semen after death', *J. Med. Eth.* (1977), 3.

Cusine, D. J., 'Status of the AID child', *SLT* (News) (1977).

Cusine, D. J., 'Womb-leasing: some legal implications', *NLJ* (1978), 128.

Da Costa, Mendes, *Studies in Canadian Family Law*, Toronto, Butterworths, 1972.

Daily Telegraph, 21 July 1984.

David, G. and Lansac, J., 'The organisation of the centers for the study and preservation of semen in France' in David and Price.

David, G. and Price, W. S., *Human Artificial Insemination and Semen Preservation*. New York, Plenum, 1980.

David, G. *et al.*, 'Results of AID for a first and succeeding pregnancies' in David and Price.

Davies, David in *The Times*, 19 July 1984.

Dawkins, R., *The Selfish Gene*. Oxford University Press, 1976, p.344.

Denning, Ld, in HL Debates, vol. 456, col. 542.

Dickens, B., *Medico-Legal Aspects of Family Law*. Toronto, Butterworths, 1979.

Dienes, C. T., 'Artificial donor insemination: perspectives on legal and social change', *Iowa LR* (1968), 54.

Dixon, R.E. and Buttram, V. C., 'Artificial insemination using donor semen: a review of 171 cases', *Fert. & Ster.* (1976), 27.

Dixon, R. E. *et. al*, 'Artificial insemination using homologous semen: a review of 158 cases', *Fert. & Ster.* (1976), 27.

Dunstan, G. R., 'Ethical issues relating to AID' in RCOG (AI).

Dunstan, G. R., 'The Moral status of the human embryo', *J. Med. Eth.* (1984), 10.

Edwards, J. H., 'Discussion opener on Mr Joyce's paper' in RCOG (AI).

Edwards, R. G., 'The current clinical and ethical situation of human conception in vitro' in Carter, C. O., ed., *Developments in Human Reproduction and their Eugenic, Ethical Implications*.

Edwards, R. G., 'Fertilisation of human eggs in vitro: morals, ethics and the law', *Quar. Rev. Biology* (1974), 49.

Edwards, R. G., 'What now for test-tube babies?', *New Scientist* (1982), 93.

Edwards, R. G. and Steptoe, P. C., *A Matter of Life*. London, Hutchinson, 1980.

Edwards, R. G. and Steptoe, P. C., 'Current status of *in vitro* fertilisation and implantation of human embryos', *Lancet* (1983), 11.

Egbert, C. L. in *Medical World*.

Eliason, R., 'Assessment of male fertility' in RCOG (AI).

Ellis, W. H., 'The socio-legal problems of artificial insemination', *Indiana Law Journal* (1953), 28.

Epstein, I., ed., *The Babylonian Talmud*. London, Soncino Press, 1938.

Finegold, W. J., *Artificial Insemination*, 2nd edn. Springfield, Ill., Thomas, 1976.

Finlay, H. A. and Bissett-Johnson, A., *Family Law in Australia*. Melbourne, Butterworths, 1972.

Finnemore, J. in *Grimes v. Grimes* (1948).

Fiscina, S., 'Information about patients: how confidential?', *Legal Medicine* (1980).

Fiumara, N. J., 'Transmission of gonorrhea by artificial insemination', *Brit. J. Venereal Diseases* (1972), 48.

Folsome, C. E., 'The status of artificial insemination: a critical review', *Am. J. Obs. & Gyn.* (1943), 45.

Foss, G. L., 'Discussion opener' in RCOG (AI).

Friedman, L. M., *A History of American Law*. New York, Simon & Schuster, 1973.

Friedmann, S., 'Artificial insemination with donor semen mixed with semen of the infertile husband', *Fert. & Ster.* (1980), 33.

Friedmann, W., *Law in a Changing Society*, 2nd edn. Harmondsworth, Penguin, 1972.

Ginzberg, L., *The Legends of the Jews*. Phila, Jewish Publication Soc. of America, 1968.

Gloag, W. M., *The Law of Contract*, 2nd edn. Edinburgh, Green, 1929.

Gloag, W. M. and Henderson, R. C., *Introduction to the Law of Scotland*, 8th edn. Edinburgh, Green, 1980.

Glover, J., *Causing Death and Saving Lives*. Harmondsworth, Penguin, 1977.

Goldstein, D. P., 'Artificial insemination by donor: status and problems' in Milunsky, A. and Annas, G. J., eds, *Genetics and the Law*. New York, Plenum Press, 1976.

Goldstein, J., Freud, A. and Solnit, A., *Beyond the Best Interests of the Child*. New York, Free Press, 1973; London, Burnett Books, 1980.

Goode, W. J., *The Family*. New York, Prentice-Hall, 1963.

Government publications:

Australia

    Artificial Conception Act 1984.

    Artificial Conception Act 1985.

    Artificial Conception Discussion Paper 1, *Human Artificial Insemination*. 1984.

    Artificial Conception Ordinance 1985.

    Artificial Conception Report on Human Artificial Insemination. 1986.

    Committee to Consider the Social, Ethical and Legal Issues Arising from In Vitro Fertilisation, *Report on Donor Gametes in IVF*. 1983.

    Infertility Medical Procedures Act 1984.

    Institute of Family Studies/Citizens Welfare Services of Victoria, *A Child is not the 'Cure' for Infertility*. National Workshop on Infertility, 1982.

    Report on the Disposition of Embryos Produced by InVitro Fertilisation. 1984.

    Report of Special Committee Appointed by the Queensland Government to Enquire into the Laws Relating to Artificial Insemination, In Vitro Fertilisation and other Related Matters. 1984.

Status of Children Amendment Act 1985.

Canada

Divorce Act.

Human Tissue Gift Act 1971.

Quebec Civil Code Act.

Royal Commission on Family and Children's Law, British Columbia, 9th Report. 1975.

Croatia: Law, 21 April 1978.

Europe

Draft Recommendation of Artificial Insemination of Human Beings. 1979.

European Committee on Legal Co-operation, 30th Meeting, 27 November–1 December 1978.

European Public Health Committee, 6th Meeting, 13–16 November 1979.

France

Civil Code.

Penal Code.

Great Britain (HMSO)

Adoption Act 1976.

Adoption (Scotland) Act 1978.

AID Children (Legal Status) Bill 1977.

Anatomy Act 1984.

'Anent Adulterie' Act 1563.

Births and Deaths Registration Act 1953.

Child Benefit Act 1975.

Children and Young Persons Act 1969.

Children's Act 1984.

Confidential Information. Working Paper no. 58 (1974); Memorandum no. 40 (1977).

Congenital Disabilities (Civil Liability) Act 1976.

Divorce (Scotland) Act 1976.

Divorce Reform Act 1969.

Divorce Statistics (England and Wales); (Scotland).

Domestic Proceedings and Magistrates Courts Act 1978.

Family Law (Scotland) Act 1985.

Family Law: illegitimacy. Working Paper no. 79, 1979; Report 1982.

Family Law: nullity of marriage. Working Paper no. 20. 1968.

Family Law Reform Act 1969.

Family Law Reform Act 1987.

Feversham Report. *Report of the Departmental Committee on Human Artificial Insemination.* Cmnd. 1105. 1960.

First Report of the Commissioners into the Law of Divorce. C. 1604. 1853.

HC Debates.

HL Debates.

Human Tissue Act 1961.

Income and Corporation Taxes Act 1970.

Inheritance (Provision for Family Dependants) Act 1975.

Law Reform (Miscellaneous Provisions) Act 1949.

Legislation on Human Infertility Services and Embryo Research: A Consultation Paper. Cm. 46. 1986.

Liability for Ante-Natal Injury. Cmnd. 5371. 1973.

Matrimonial and Family Proceedings Act 1984.

Matrimonial Causes Act 1973.

Matrimonial Proceedings (Children) Act 1958.

Medical Act 1983.

Mental Health Act 1983.

Mental Health (Scotland) Act 1984.

National Health Service (Venereal Disease) Regulations 1974.

Nullity of Marriage Act 1971.

Population Trends, no. 14 (1978); no. 30 (1982); no. 44 (1986).

Registration of Births, Deaths and Marriages (Scotland) Act 1965.

Report of Voluntary Licensing Authority for Human In Vitro Fertilisation and Embryology. 1986.

Report on Injuries to Unborn Children. Cmnd. 5709. 1974.

Royal Commission on Civil Liability and Compensation for Personal Injuries. Cmnd. 7054–1. 1974.

Royal Commission on Marriage and Divorce. Cmnd. 9678. 1956.

Social Trends. 1986.

Statement on in vitro fertilisation and embryo transfer. 3 September 1982.

Surrogacy Arrangements Act 1985.

The Use of Foetuses and Foetal Material for Research. Peel Report. 1972.

Warnock. *Report of the Committee of Inquiry into Human Fertilisation and Embryology*. Cmnd. 9314. 1984.

Israel

Ministry of Health Rules Concerning the Administration of Sperm Banks and Directives for the Performance of Artificial Insemination. 1979.

Italy: Penal Code.

Netherlands: Civil Code.

New Zealand: New Zealand Compensation Act 1974.

Portugal: Civil Code.

Slovenia: Law, 21 April 1977.

South Africa: Anatomical Donations and Post Mortem Examination Act 24 (1970).

BIBLIOGRAPHY 247

Switzerland
Civil Code.
Guidelines on Medical Ethics Concerning Artificial Insemination, 17
November 1981.
West Germany: Civil Code.
USA
Ethics Advisory Board, *Health Education and Welfare Support of
Research involving Human in Vitro Fertilisation and Embryo
Transfer*. Washington, DC, 1979.
Ethics Advisory Board, *New Support of Research involving Human
in vitro Fertilisation and Embryo Transfer*. 1979.
Indiana House Bill 350 (1949).
Law Reform Commission (Saskatchewan), *Tentative Proposals for
a Human Artificial Insemination Act*. 1981.
Minnesota House Bills 1090, 1091, 1092 (1949).
New York City Health Code 1959, *Artificial Human Insemination*.
New York Domestic Relations Law 1969.
New York Senate Bills 745 (1948); 772 (1949); 579 (1950); 493
(1951).
Ohio Senate Bill 93 (1955).
Report of Ethics Advisory Board, May 1979.
State Legislation on legitimacy of AI children: see list in ch. 8,
n.56.
Statistical Abstracts 1985. Dept. of Commerce, Bureau of the
Census.
*Sub-Committee on Children and Youth of the Committee on Labor and
Public Welfare*, 94th Congress, 28–9 April 1975.
Uniform Marriage and Divorce Act.
Uniform Parentage Act 1973.
Virginia Senate Bill 199 (1948).
Wisconsin Assembly Bill 407 (1949).
Graveson, R. H., *Status in the Common Law*. London, Athlone Press,
1953.
Greenway, Harry, in HC Debates, vol. 73, col. 531.
Greer, L. J. in *Hall v. Brooklands Auto-Racing Club* (1933).
Guardian, 16 April 1984; 21 July 1984; 9 March 1986.
Gurdon, J. B. and Laskey, R. A., 'The transplantation of nuclei
from single cultured cells', *J. Embryology and Experimental
Morphology* (1970), 24.
Guttmacher, A. F., 'Artificial insemination', *De Paul Law Rev.* (1969),
18.
Guttmacher, A. F., 'The role of artificial insemination in the treat-
ment of human sterility', *Bull. NY Academy of Science* (1943), 119.
Guttmacher, A. F., 'The role of artificial insemination in the treat-
ment of sterility', *Obs. & Gyn. Survey* (1960), 15.

Hahlo, H. R., 'Some legal aspects of human artificial insemination', *SALJ*, 74.

Hahlo, H. R., *The South African Law of Husband and Wife*. Cape Town, Juta.

Hahlo, H. R. and Kahn, E., *The Union of South Africa: the development of its laws and constitution*. London, Stevens, 1965.

Haldane, J. B. S., 'Biological possibilities in the next 10 000 years' in Wolstenholme, G., ed., *Man and his Future*. London, Churchill, 1963.

Halsbury, Earl of, in HL Debates, vol. 456, col. 558.

Haman, J. O., 'Therapeutic donor insemination: a review of 440 cases', *Calif. Med.* (1959), 90.

Hamilton, N. in *Medical World*.

Hard, A. D., 'Artificial impregnation', *Medical World* (1909), 27.

Harris, C. C., *The Family*. London, Allen & Unwin, 1979.

Harris, L. E., 'Artificial insemination and surrogate motherhood', *Williamette LR* (1981), 17.

Harrison, R. G. and de Boer, C. H., *Sex and Infertility*. London, Academic Press, 1977.

Hart, H. L. A. and Honore, A. M., *Causation in the Law*. Oxford, Clarendon Press, 1959.

Heape, W., 'Preliminary note on the transplantation and growth of mammalian ova within a uterine foster mother', *Proc. Royal Society (B. Biological Sciences)* (1890), 48, pp.457–8.

Hill, A. M., 'Experiences with artificial insemination', *Aust. & NZ J. Obs. & Gyn.* (1970), 10.

Hill, G. B., ed., *Boswell's Life of Johnson*. Oxford, Clarendon Press, 1887.

Holder, A. R., *Medical Malpractice Law*, 2nd edn. New York, Wiley, 1978.

Home, E., 'An account of the dissection of a hermaphrodite dog' in *Phil. Trans. Royal Society*, 18.

'Human artificial insemination', *BMJ* (1973), 2, Supp. (7 April).

Human Artificial Insemination. Report of the Archbishop of Canterbury's Commission. SPCK, 1948.

'Human embryo banks proposed', *The Times*, 28 January 1982.

Human Fertilisation and Embryology. London, Royal Society, 1983.

'Human reproduction: regulated progress or damned interference', *Lancet* (1984), 2.

Hume, John, in HC Debates, vol. 73, col. 569.

Hume's Lectures, (1766–1822) I. Stair Society (1939), vol. 5.

Iglesias, T., 'In vitro fertilisation: the major issues', *J. Med. Eth.* (1984), 10.

Innes, C. J. in *Bell v. Bell* (1909).

'Interim report on human in vitro fertilisation and embryo replacement and transfer', *BMJ* (1983), 286.

In Vitro Fertilisation: morality and public policy. Abbots Langley, Catholic Information Services, 1983.

IPPF, *Handbook on Infertility*. London, 1979.

Jacob, J., ed., *Speller's Law Relating to Hospitals and Kindred Institutions*, 6th edn. London, H. K. Lewis, 1978.

Jacobs, R. S. and Luedtke, J. P., 'Social and legal aspects of human artificial insemination', *Wisconsin LR* (1965), 40.

Jacquard, A. and Schoevaeri, D., 'Artificial insemination and consanguinity' in David and Price.

Johnston, I., 'The donor' in Wood.

Jones, A. and Bodmer, W. F., *Our Future Inheritance: choice or chance?* Oxford University Press, 1976.

Joyce, D., 'Recruitment, selection and matching of donors' in RCOG (AI).

Kardiman, S., 'Artificial insemination in the Talmud', *Harofe Haivri: Hebrew Medical Journal* (1950), 2.

Keane, N. and Breo, D., *The Surrogate Mother*. New York, Everest House, 1981.

Kelly, H. A., 'Kinship, incest and the dictates of law', *Am. J. Juris* (1969), 14.

Kerr, M. and Templeton, A., 'Selection and counselling of recipients' in RCOG (AI).

Kilbrandon, Ld, in Ciba.

Klayman, E. T., 'Therapeutic impregnation: prognosis of a lawyer – diagnosis of a legislature', *Univ. Cincinnati LR* (1970), 39.

Kilbanoff, E. B., 'Genealogical information in adoption', *Family Law Quarterly* (1977), 11.

Klopper, A. I., Univ. Aberdeen. Personal communication.

Klugman, S. J., 'Therapeutic donor insemination', *Fert. & Ster.* (1954), 5.

Klugman, S. J. and Kaufman, S. A., *Infertility in Women*. Phila, Davis, 1966.

Krause, H. D., *Family Law: cases and materials*, 2nd edn. St Paul, Minn., West Pub., 1983.

Krause, H. D., *Illegitimacy: law and social policy*. New York, Bobbs Merrill, 1971.

Kritchevsky, B., 'The unmarried woman's right to artificial insemination: a call for expanded definition of family', *Harvard Women's Law Journal* (1981), 4.

Kuhse, H. and Singer, P., 'The moral status of the embryo' in Walters and Singer.

Lancet (1984), 1, editorial.

Lang, D., 'Artificial insemination: legitimate or illegitimate', *McCall's Magazine* (May 1955).

Leach, W. B., 'Perpetuities in the atomic age: the sperm bank and the fertile decedent', *ABAJ* (1962), 48.

Lebech, P. E., 'Present status of AID and sperm banks in Denmark' in David and Price.

Lebech, P. E. and Detlefsen, G., 'Artificial insemination with frozen spermatozoa: results from 1967 to 1978' in David and Price.

Ledenburg, J., 'Experimental genetics and human evolution', *Bulletin of the Atomic Scientists* (1966).

Leeton, J. F., 'The development and demand for AID in Australia' in Wood.

Levisohn, A. A., 'Dilemma in parenthood', *J. For. Med.* (1957), 4.

Longford, Ld, in HL Debates, vol. 456, col. 575.

Los Angeles Times, 29 February 1980.

Lothian, Marquess of, in HL Debates, vol. 456, col. 566.

Loveset, J., 'Artificial insemination: the attitude of patients in Norway', *Fert. & Ster.* (1951), 2.

McIntosh, T. M. in *Medical World*.

McLean, S., 'The right to reproduce' in Campbell *et al.*

McNair, J. in *Bolam v. Friern Hospital Management Committee* (1957).

McNeil, I. R., *Contracts*. New York, Foundation Press, 1978.

McTaggart, L., 'How I sold – and almost bought a baby', *Sunday New York News Magazine*, 13 April 1975.

Mahoney, J., *Bioethics and Belief*. London, Sheed & Ward, 1984.

Marina, S., 'The first sperm bank in Spain: organisation and first year results' in David and Price.

Mason, J. K. and McCall-Smith, A. A., *Law and Medical Ethics*. London, Butterworths, 1983.

Mattei, A. *et al.*, 'The male factor in AID requests' in David and Price.

Meston, Ld, in HL Debates, vol. 456, col. 583.

Milunsky, A. and Annas, G. J., eds, *Genetics and the Law*. New York, Plenum Press, 1976.

Milverton, Ld, in HL Debates, vol. 456, col. 579.

Montemuro, J. in *Manbeck v. Manbeck*.

'Moppets on the market: the problem of unregulated adoptions', *Yale Law Journal* (1950), 59.

Moser, W., 'Population genetics and AID' in David and Price.

Muasher, S. J. *et al.*, 'Benefits and risks of multiple transfer with in vitro fertilisation', *Lancet* (1984), II.

Muller, H. J., 'Genetic progress by voluntarily conducted germinal choice' in Wolstenholme, ed., *Man and his Future*.

Newill, R., *Infertile Marriage*. Harmondsworth, Penguin, 1974.

Newth, C. H. in *Medical World*.

Newton, J. R., 'Current status of AI in clinical practice' in RCOG (AI).

New York Post, 28 March 1955.

New York Times, 11 December 1985.

Norwich, Bp of, in HL Debates, vol. 456, col. 553.

Paisley, Revd Ian, HC Debates, vol. 73, col. 554.

Philipp, E., *Childlessness: its causes and what to do about them*. London, Arrow, 1975.

Pilcher, J. in *Cowen v. Cowen* (1946).

Ploscowe, M., 'The place of law in medico-moral problems: a legal view', *NYULR* (1956), 31.

Ploscowe, M., *Sex and the Law*. New York, Prentice-Hall, 1951.

Portnoy, L., 'Artificial insemination (AID): experiences with its use in eighty barren marriages', *Fert. & Ster.* (1956), 7.

Portuando, J. A. and Echanojaurequi, A. D., 'Human semen bank at the Spanish Social Security Hospital' in David and Price.

Prosser, W. L., *Handbook of the Law of Torts*, 6th edn. St Paul, Minn., West Pub., 1976.

Prys-Davies, Ld, in HL Debates, vol. 456, col. 586.

Quinlivan, W. L. G. and Sullivan, M., 'The immunologic effects of husband's semen on donor spermatozoa during mixed insemination', *Fert. & Ster.* (1977), 24.

Rachels, J., 'Active and passive euthanasia', *NEJM* (1975), 292.

Rawlinson of Ewell, Ld, in HL Debates, vol. 456, cols 555–6.

Raynor, L., *The Adopted Child Comes of Age*. London, Allen & Unwin, 1980.

RCOG (AI): *Artificial Insemination*. Proc. of 4th College Study Group of RCOG. 1976.

Reading, Marquess of, in HL Debates, vol. 456, cols 535–7.

Report of RCOG Ethics Committee on In Vitro Fertilisation and Embryo Replacement or Transfer. 1983.

Report of RCOG Working Party on Further Specialisations within Obstetrics and Gynaecology. 1982.

'Research related to human fertilisation and embryology' (1982), *BMJ*, 285.

Research Related to Human Fertilisation and Embryology. London, MRC, 1982.

Rheinstein, M., *Marriage Stability, Divorce and the Law*. Univ. Chicago Press, 1972.

Rice, C. E., 'AID: an heir of controversy', *Notre Dame Lawyer* (1959), 34.

Rioux, J. E. and Ackman, C. D. F., 'Artificial insemination and sperm banks: the Canadian experience' in David and Price.

Robertson of Oakbridge, Ld, in HL Debates, vol. 456, col. 567.

Rohleder, H., *Test-Tube Babies: a history of the artificial impregnation of human beings*. New York, Panurge Press, 1934.

Root, Chas A., Senator in Minnesota. Letter to the author.

Rorvik, David, *In his Image: the cloning of a man*. New York, Lippincott, 1978.

Rosner, F., *Studies in Torah Judaism: modern medicine and Jewish Law*. New York, Yeshiva Univ., 1972.

Rossi, Sir Hugh, in HC Debates, vol. 73, col. 562.

Rowson, L. E. A. and Morr, R. M., 'Non-surgical transfer of cow eggs', *J. Reprod. & Fert*. (1966), 11.

Rubin, B., 'Psychological aspects of human artificial insemination', *Arch. Gen. Psychiat*. (1965), 13.

Russell, B., *Marriage and Morals*. London, Allen & Unwin 1961.

Saltoun, Lady, in HL Debates, vol. 456, col. 563.

Sants, H. J., 'Genealogical bewilderment in children with substitute parents', *Brit. J. Med. Psych*. (1964), 37.

Sappideen, C., 'Life after death – sperm banks, wills and perpetuities', *Aus. LJ* (1979), 53.

Saunders, D. M., 'The assessment of the infertile couple for AID' in Wood.

Schellen, A. M. C. M., *Artificial Insemination in the Human*. Amsterdam, Elsevier, 1957.

Schoysman, R., 'Problems of selecting donors for AI', *J. Med. Eth*. (1975), 1.

Schoysman, R. and Schoysman-Deboeck, A., 'Present status of donor insemination in Belgium' in David and Price.

'Schweizerische Aerztezeitung', *Bulletin des Medecins Suisses* (1982), 62, no. 11.

Scotsman, 4 March 1986.

Scott, R., *The Body as Property*. London, Allen Lane, 1981.

Seashore, R. T., 'Artificial impregnation', *Minn. Med*. (1933), 21.

Sergeant, D. A., 'Legal status of artificial insemination: a need for policy formulation', *Drake LR* (1970), 19.

Seymour, F. I. and Koerner, A., 'Artificial insemination, present status in the USA as shown by a recent survey', *JAMA* (1941), 116.

Shell, Thurston A., 'Artificial insemination – legal and related problems', *U. Fla. LR* (1955), 8.

Sherman, J. K., 'Historical synopsis of human semen cryobanking' in David and Price.

Sherman, J. K., 'Synopsis of the use of human frozen semen since 1964: state of the art of human semen banking', *Fert. & Ster*. (1973), 24.

Sherman, J. K. and Rosenfeld, J., 'Importance of frozen-stored human semen in the spread of gonorrhea', *Fert. & Ster.* (1975), 26.

Sherman, J. S., 'People v. Sorensen: artificial insemination gives birth to legal problems in California', *California Western LR* (1968), 4.

Singer, P. and Wells, D., *The Reproductive Revolution: new ways of making babies.* Oxford University Press, 1984.

Slome, J., 'Artificial insemination by donor', *BMJ* (1973), 2.

Slovenko, R., *Sexual Behaviour and the Law.* Ill., Thomas, 1965.

Smith, George P. II, 'Through a test tube darkly: artificial insemination and the law', *Michigan* (1968–69), 67.

Smith, R. S. and Tagatz, G. E., 'Acute gonorrhea after artificial insemination', *Fert. & Ster.* (1976), 27.

Snowden, R. and Mitchell, G. D., *The Artificial Family: a consideration of artificial insemination by donor.* London, Allen & Unwin, 1981.

Snowden, R., Mitchell, G. D. and Snowden, E. M., *Artificial Reproduction: a social investigation.* London, Allen & Unwin, 1983.

Speichinger, J. P. and Maddox, J. J., 'Homologous artificial insemination and oligospermia', *Fert. & Ster.* (1976), 27.

Stair, *The Institutions of the Law of Scotland*, 5th edn, ed. More, J. S. (Edinburgh, Bell & Bradfute, 1832), III.

Stangel, J. J., *Fertility and Conception: an essential guide for childless couples.* London, Paddington Press, 1979.

Steinberger, E. and Smith, K. D., 'Artificial insemination with fresh or frozen semen', *JAMA* (1973), 223.

Steptoe, P. C. (1984). Paper given at BMA Scientific Meeting, Cambridge (April).

Sulewski, J. M. *et al.*, 'A longitudinal analysis of artificial insemination with donor semen', *Fert. & Ster.* (1978), 29.

Sunday Times, 4 June 1978; 21 August 1983; 13 January 1985; 26 April 1986.

Swinbanks, D., 'Gender selection sparks row', *Nature* (1986), 321.

Swiss Academy of Medical Sciences, *Guidelines* (1981).

The Times, 28 March 1896; 12 May 1960; 2 September 1978; 7 February 1984; 18 June 1984; 11, 21, 23, 25, 31 July 1984; 3 August 1984; 25 October 1984; 20, 26 November 1984; 7, 23 January 1985; 30 July 1985; 14 September 1985; 21 January 1986; 24 April 1986; 26 June 1986; 2, 4 July 1986.

Thies, W. D., 'A look to the future: property rights and the posthumously conceived child', *Trusts and Estates* (1971), 110.

Thompson, C. M., 'The legal consequences of artificial insemination in South Dakota', *South Dakota L. R.* (1968), 13.

Titmus, R., *The Gift of Relationship.* New York, Pantheon, 1971.

Traina, V., 'Artificial insemination and semen banks in Italy' in David and Price.

Tranmire, Ld, in HL Debates, vol. 456, col. 574.

Treitel, G. H., *The Law of Contract*, 6th edn. London, Stevens, 1979.

Triselotis, J., 'Identity and adoption', *Child Adoption* (1974), 78.

Triselotis, J., *In Search of Origins: the experience of adopted people.* London, Routledge, 1973.

Trounson, A. *et al.*, 'Pregnancy established in an infertile patient after transfer of a donated embryo fertilised in vitro', *BMJ* (1983), 286.

Veatch, R. M., *Case Studies in Medical Ethics.* Cambridge, Mass., Harvard Univ. Press, 1977.

Verkauf, B. S., 'Artificial insemination: progress, polemics and confusion – an appraisal of current medico-legal status', *Houston LR* (1966), 3.

Wadlington, W., 'Artificial insemination: the dangers of a poorly kept secret', *North Western Univ. LR* (1970), 64.

Walker, D. M., *The Law of Delict in Scotland*, 2nd edn. Edinburgh, Green, 1982.

Walker, D. M., *Principles of Scottish Private Law*, 3rd edn. Oxford University Press, 1983.

Wall Street Journal, 24 June 1971.

Walters, W. and Singer, P., *Test-Tube Babies: a guide to moral questions and future possibilities.* Melbourne, Oxford University Press, 1982.

Wangard, R. E., 'Artificial insemination and the law', *Univ. Ill. Law Forum* (1968).

Weisman, A. I., 'Selection of donors for use in artificial insemination', *West. J. Surg.* (1942), 50.

Weinstock, N., 'Artificial insemination: the problem and the solution', *Family Law Quarterly* (1971), 5.

Westermarck, E., *The History of Human Marriage.* London, Macmillan, 1921.

Westermarck, E., *The Origin and Development of the Moral Ideas.* London, Macmillan, 1906–8.

Wheatley, Ld, in *MacLennan v. MacLennan* (1958).

'Woman having baby for transsexual sister', *The Times*, 17 January 1981.

Wood, C., *Artificial Insemination by Donor.* Melbourne, Monash University Press, 1980.

Yanigamachi, R. *et al.*, 'The use of zona-free animal ova as a test system for the assessment of the fertilisation capacity of human spermatozoa', *Biological Reproduction* (1976), 15.

Index

and impotence, distinction
  between 26
male 3, 6–7, 109–10
solutions to 8–10
statistics 5
statutory licensing authority on
  173–4
intelligence 102
International Code of Ethics of the
  World Medical Association 74
International Planned Parenthood
  Federation 92
In Vitro Fertilisation and Embryo
  Replacement or Transfer,
  Report on 130
in vitro fertilization (IVF) 3, 10, 11,
  17–18, 130–41, 176, 185, 186
action by child 132–3
action by parents 133–4
in Australia 140–1
doctor's involvement in 167–8
and egg donation 129–30, 141–2
and embryonic biopsy 190
in UK 137–9
in USA 139–40
in vivo fertilization 185

Jacobi, Ludwig 12
Jews 103
Johnson, Dr Samuel 40
*Journal of the American Medical
  Association* 14

Karminski 37
Kilbrandon, Lord 67
Kitson v. Playfair 76
Klinefelter's Syndrome 24
Koerner 14, 17

Lancet 162, 179, 197
laparoscopy 112, 113, 131
Latey, Mr Justice 150, 197
'lavage' 176
Law Commission (England and
  Wales) 29, 77, 106, 174, 175
Law Reform Commission of New
  South Wales, Report of 203–5
Law Reform Commission of
  Ontario 198

Leeton, J. F., *Artificial Insemination
  by Donor* 15
Legal Cooperation, European
  Committee on (CDCJ) 94
legitimacy *see* illegitimacy
lesbians 108, 118, 119
Lesch-Nyham Syndrome 99
Lovallo v. NJ State Registrar 84
Lushington, Dr 27

McCall's Magazine 17
McComb, Justice 46, 55
MacLennan v. MacLennan 28, 46, 47,
  49
Macnaughton, Professor M. C. 199
maintenance of AID children 35,
  52–6
Marsham, Lady 195
Meacher, Michael 196
Medical World 13
menopause 7
miscarriages 199
mongolism *see* Down's Syndrome
Mosaic Law 45
MRC 137, 138, 174, 185
Muller, Dr Hermann 43
multiple sclerosis 154
mumps 7
muscular dystrophy 199

National Centre for Surrogate
  Parenting 196
National Health and Medical
  Research Council of Australia
  181
National Health Service (NHS) 76,
  103, 172, 173, 176, 177, 195
Nature 132, 179, 197
necrospermia 6
New South Wales Law Reform
  Commission 202
New York City Health Code 75, 82,
  101
New York Post 17
News Chronicle 17
nucleus substitution 186, 190–2
nurturing father 4
nurturing mother 3–4, 144